Wall Pilates for Seniors

The Ultimate 28-Day Challenge with illustrated Workouts for Modern Woman and Senior Seeking Strength and Flexibility

DENISE KELLEY

2

DENISE KELLEY

SPECIAL BONUS!

Want this bonus book for free?

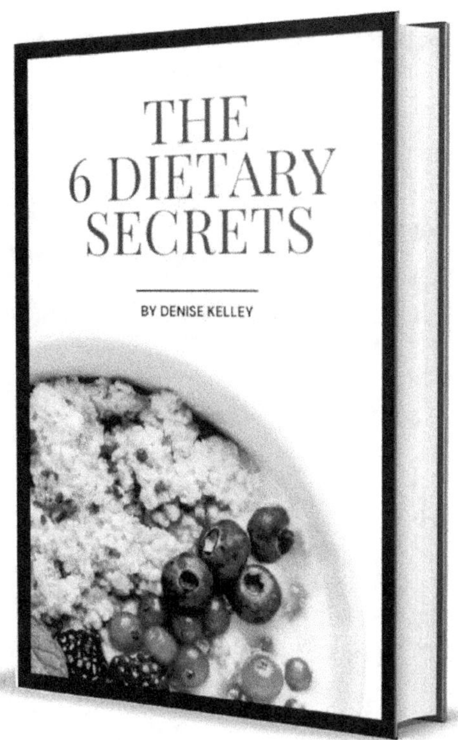

Get FREE, unlimited access to it and all of my new books by joining the Fan Base!

Scan the QR Code to join!

Table of Contents

Introduction: A Personal Invitation to the Wall Pilates Journey

Greetings, wonderful women! I'm overjoyed to invite you into the world of "Wall Pilates for Seniors." I'm Denise Kelley, not just your guide but a living testament to the incredible impact of Wall Pilates. Picture me not as an author but as someone who's walked the Wall Pilates path, experiencing a profound transformation.

Years back, as the echoes of aging grew louder, Wall Pilates entered my life, becoming a catalyst for remarkable change. I faced doubts, but through its gentle yet powerful movements, I discovered strength, flexibility, and joy.

Now, I stand taller, move gracefully, and radiate vitality. Wall Pilates isn't just an exercise; it's a sanctuary where I reclaimed control and embraced the beauty of time passing!

In the coming chapters, we'll unravel Wall Pilates, from stretch fundamentals to breath work, making it accessible. This isn't just movement; it's understanding your body's language fluently.

Let's talk about navigating this journey. The rules and instructions ahead are your personal GPS through Wall Pilates. From warm-up to cool-down, I'll guide every step, ensuring a delightful process and maximum benefits.

But let's move beyond technicalities; let's delve into the heart—the personal stories. Picture Maria, a vibrant grandmother finding solace, or Jessica, a busy professional striking a balance. Imagine Sarah, a retiree joyfully stretching against the wall, or Lisa, a mother seamlessly incorporating Wall Pilates, gaining energy and resilience.

These stories illuminate Wall Pilates' universal appeal, transcending age, background, or fitness level—a journey for everyone. Whether a fitness enthusiast or a novice, Wall Pilates welcomes you. Its adaptability suits diverse lifestyles.

As you delve into the chapters, know you're not alone. Together, we'll explore the transformative magic of Wall Pilates, embracing the richness of every age and background.

Now, let's explore how to make the most of Wall Pilates for Seniors.

How to Get the Most from This Pilates Challenge

Embarking on this Wall Pilates journey isn't just about exercises; it's about creating an environment that fosters focus, consistency, and well-being. Here's a guide to making the most of this transformative journey!

Establishing a Routine:
For beginners, consistency is key. Engage in Wall Pilates at least twice a week, with the sweet spot often being three times. While daily practice is acceptable, recovery is crucial. Muscles build during recovery, so be patient as Wall Pilates unfolds gradually.

Embracing Recovery:
Amidst the excitement, remember that muscles repair during recovery. Daily practice should be mindful of recovery. Again, patience is crucial; Wall Pilates unfolds gradually, like a delicate flower.

Navigating Challenges for Maximum Gains:
Expect challenges, especially with daunting exercises. Paradoxically, these challenges yield significant benefits. Embrace difficulty as an opportunity for growth – each stretch is a step towards enhanced strength and flexibility.

Consistency and Progress:
A consistent routine is your compass. It tracks progress and measures achievements. As Wall Pilates becomes a part of your routine, witness the evolution of strength, flexibility, and overall well-being. Keep a journal – it's a testament to your commitment.

Adaptability and Growth:
Flexibility is not just about stretching muscles; it's also about adapting your routine. As you grow proficient, adjust and expand. Modify exercises, add variations, and explore Wall Pilates' vast possibilities. Your journey is dynamic, and so should be your practice.

In conclusion, let this book be your companion. Embrace the recommended frequency, honor recovery, and savor the gradual unfolding of results. Navigate challenges, establish consistency, and remember, Wall Pilates is not just exercise – it's a lifestyle, a journey, and a celebration of your strength and resilience. Let the transformative odyssey begin!

Excitedly,
Your Denise.

Chapter 1: The Wall Pilates - Health Boost, Benefits, and Motivation

Welcome to the realm of Pilates, a distinctive low-impact exercise method designed to fortify muscles and enhance posture and flexibility. Typically conducted in a class setting, these sessions span 45 minutes to an hour, emphasizing unhurried, precise movements synchronized with your breath. While core muscles take the spotlight, engagements for arms, glutes, and lower legs are also incorporated.

Enter Wall Pilates, a unique variation leveraging your body weight and the resistance a wall provides to amplify muscle engagement and flexibility. Different from traditional Pilates, this variation requires no specialized equipment. Movements unfold gradually and with control, using the wall as a reliable support to stretch and tone muscles. So, what sets Wall Pilates apart? Let's dissect the elements that make it stand out:

Utilization of the Wall:
The defining feature of Wall Pilates is the integration of a wall as both a support and resistance tool. This innovative addition expands the range of exercises, making Wall Pilates adaptable to diverse fitness levels.

Increased Resistance and Intensity:
The wall elevates the challenge for your muscles by introducing an extra layer of resistance. This heightened intensity results in a workout that surpasses traditional mat-based Pilates, fostering more significant strength gains and calorie burn.

Improved Alignment and Posture:
The wall acts as a reliable guide, ensuring proper alignment and posture throughout exercises. Emphasizing correct form minimizes injury risks and engages the right muscle groups, promoting enhanced posture and body awareness.

Greater Balance and Stability:
The wall becomes a steadfast ally during balance exercises, providing support that simplifies maintaining stability while executing movements that might pose challenges on a mat or other Pilates equipment. This added stability allows you to concentrate on core engagement and overall balance.

Variety of Exercises:
Wall Pilates weaves together a rich tapestry of exercises, drawing inspiration from traditional mat Pilates, reformer Pilates, and even yoga. This diversity keeps the

workouts dynamic, reducing the risk of monotony and encouraging sustained commitment.

Accessibility:
A noteworthy aspect of Wall Pilates is its flexibility in practice settings. Whether at home, in a gym, or at a specialized studio, all required is a sturdy wall and a mat. This accessibility makes Wall Pilates an inclusive option for those without access to elaborate Pilates equipment.

Navigating the Challenges of Wall Pilates

While Wall Pilates offers a myriad of benefits, it's essential to acknowledge and unpack the complexities that can make it challenging:

Increased Resistance:
The wall introduces an extra layer of resistance, intensifying the demands on your muscles. This heightened resistance necessitates increased effort, making Wall Pilates more challenging than its mat-based counterpart.

Higher Intensity:
Wall Pilates demands heightened focus and muscle activation by incorporating strength, flexibility, and balance exercises. This elevated intensity sets it apart, presenting a more challenging workout than other exercise forms.

Emphasis on Proper Form and Alignment:
Maintaining correct form and alignment becomes paramount in Wall Pilates. Ensuring the engagement of the right muscle groups and executing movements correctly may pose challenges, especially for beginners or those with limited body awareness. We will address this crucial aspect in each one of the poses we will do together!

Core Engagement:
As with traditional Pilates, Wall Pilates significantly emphasizes activating and strengthening core muscles. Effectively engaging the core, especially while maintaining proper alignment and executing complex movements, can be a formidable challenge.

Learning Curve:
As with any novel exercise routine, there's a learning curve associated with mastering Wall Pilates. Familiarizing yourself with the exercises, understanding how to leverage the wall for support and resistance, and developing the necessary strength and flexibility may take time.

Individual Fitness Level:
The difficulty of Wall Pilates varies based on your current fitness level. Beginners or those with lower fitness levels may initially find Wall Pilates more challenging. However, as strength, flexibility, and body awareness improve, the exercises become more manageable.

Benefits Unveiled

The wall introduces an additional resistance layer, fostering muscle strength and bolstering stability. Particularly advantageous for beginners, adults, or seniors, Wall Pilates facilitates quickly attaining challenging positions, providing a comforting sense of security. Let's explore its main benefits.

1. Enhanced Core Strength:
Wall Pilates emerged as a remedy in an era marked by sedentary lifestyles. It effectively strengthens the the abdominal muscles[1] and those in your back and sides, promoting better posture and alleviating issues like back pain. The wall stabilizes your spine, enabling a concentrated engagement of deep abdominal muscles — a feat often challenging with mat Pilates alone.

2. Improved Muscular Endurance and Strength:
Muscular endurance, crucial for repetitive contractions against resistance, is fortified through Wall Pilates' deliberate and controlled movements. The wall introduces extra resistance, facilitating the augmentation of exercise intensity without conventional weights, a fundamental principle in progressive overload.

3. Flexibility Enhancement:
Renowned for its muscle-building and flexibility synergy, this discipline moves further with Wall Pilates. The wall becomes a tool to deepen stretches, expanding your range of motion and enhancing flexibility.

4. Low-Impact Exercise:
Stepping away from the strain on joints associated with high-impact activities, Wall Pilates offers a low-impact alternative. This makes it an ideal choice for individuals contending with joint pain or recuperating from injuries. Its application in rehabilitation programs underscores its capacity to improve core strength, flexibility, and muscular endurance without exacerbating common stress.

---

[1] https://www.sciencedirect.com/science/article/abs/pii/S1360859220302138

5. Improved Posture and Alignment:
Wall Pilates places a premium on maintaining proper alignment throughout exercises and correcting posture imbalances. The wall serves as a guide, ensuring alignment of the spine, shoulders, and hips, resulting in improved posture and diminished risk of injury in daily activities.

6. Enhanced Balance and Stability:
The wall, providing a stable surface, simplifies maintaining balance during exercises. This, in turn, enhances overall balance and stability over time, both within the studio and beyond.

7. Greater Flexibility:
Incorporating stretching and lengthening movements, Wall Pilates contributes to increased flexibility in muscles and joints. The wall acts as a support system, facilitating the safe deepening of stretches and access to a broader range of motion.

8. Higher Calorie Burn:
The added resistance prompts muscles to work harder, leading to a higher calorie burn than mat-based Pilates. This characteristic positions Wall Pilates as an effective weight loss or maintenance option.

Additional Benefits of Wall Pilates

Beyond the core benefits, Wall Pilates unfolds a spectrum of advantages contributing to its effectiveness:

Better Pain Management:
By improving posture and strengthening muscles, particularly in the lower back, neck, and shoulders, Wall Pilates aids in pain alleviation[2]. The wall support fosters proper alignment, reducing joint strain and alleviating discomfort.

Better Cognitive Functioning:
Engaging in Wall Pilates triggers the release of endorphins, enhancing cognitive function and mental clarity[3]. Breath control and mind-body awareness in the practice reduce stress and elevate concentration[4].

---

[2] https://www.ncbi.nlm.nih.gov/pmc/articles/PMC6581086/
[3] https://www.mdpi.com/1422-0067/22/1/338
[4] https://www.researchgate.net/publication/271671902_Pilates_and_Mindfulness_A_Qualitative_Study

Improved Athletic Performance:
Athletes stand to gain from Wall Pilates, as it enhances functional strength, balance, and flexibility – crucial elements for optimal performance [5]. Improved core strength and stability translate to better power transfer, increased agility, and reduced injury risk.

Bone Health:
Weight-bearing exercises in Wall Pilates contribute to increased bone density, mitigating age-related bone mass loss. This positively impacts overall bone health and lowers the risk of osteoporosis and fractures [6].

Mood Boost:
Wall Pilates, like other forms of exercise, stimulates endorphin release [7]. The mindful movement, breath control, and physical exertion collectively reduce stress, anxiety, and negative emotions, leaving you energized and positive.

Versatility and Adaptability:
Wall Pilates offers exercises adaptable to different fitness levels and goals. The wall serves as both support for beginners and a tool to intensify exercises for advanced practitioners. This adaptability renders Wall Pilates effective for people of varying ages and abilities!

Wall Pilates Facilitates Weight Loss

For those on a weight loss journey, Wall Pilates emerges as a potent ally, owing to the following factors:

Higher Intensity:
The wall's additional resistance elevates exercise intensity, demanding more effort and resulting in a higher calorie burn. This intensified workout contributes to effective weight loss.

Increased Muscle Mass:
Wall Pilates focuses on building lean muscle mass. As muscle mass increases, the resting metabolic rate rises, translating to more calories burned at rest – a key factor in weight loss.

[5] https://www.ncbi.nlm.nih.gov/pmc/articles/PMC3666467/
[6] https://journals.plos.org/plosone/article?id=10.1371/journal.pone.0251391
[7] https://www.ncbi.nlm.nih.gov/pmc/articles/PMC4449495/

Full-Body Workout:
Comprehensively targeting multiple muscle groups, including core, upper body, and lower body, Wall Pilates ensures a thorough workout. This full-body engagement increases calorie expenditure per session, aiding in weight loss.

Improved Metabolism:
Regular Wall Pilates sessions can boost metabolism, enhancing the body's calorie-burning efficiency. This increased metabolism supports weight loss by elevating the overall calorie burn throughout the day.

Reduced Stress:
The mindful nature of Wall Pilates, coupled with breath control, contributes to stress reduction. Lower stress levels positively impact weight loss, as stress is often connected to weight gain and unhealthy eating habits.

In closing, while Wall Pilates poses its challenges, its undeniable effectiveness, adaptability, and versatility make it a rewarding and transformative exercise method. With consistent practice and proper guidance, Wall Pilates becomes a dynamic component of your fitness journey, paving the way for stronger health and well-being.

Practical Strategies for Success

Embarking on your Wall Pilates journey is not just about physical exertion; it's a commitment to your well-being. To ensure your motivation remains steadfast, consider incorporating these practical strategies into your routine:

1. Set Achievable Goals:
Begin your Wall Pilates venture by defining clear and achievable goals. Whether mastering a specific move, enhancing flexibility, or completing a set number of sessions per week, having tangible objectives provides a roadmap for your progress. Break down greater goals into smaller, more manageable milestones – celebrating these victories fuels your motivation.

2. Track Your Progress:
Nothing fuels motivation quite like witnessing tangible progress. Keep a dedicated journal or utilize fitness tracking apps to record your achievements, no matter how small. From improved posture to conquering challenging exercises, tracking your journey highlights your growth and serves as a visual reminder of your dedication.

3. Cultivate a Supportive Community:
Surround yourself with like-minded people who share your passion for Wall Pilates. Whether joining a local class, engaging in online forums, or enlisting a workout buddy, a supportive community fosters encouragement and camaraderie. Sharing experiences, challenges, and triumphs with others makes the journey more enjoyable and provides a network of motivation during moments of wavering determination.

4. Celebrate Milestones:
Acknowledge and celebrate your achievements along the way. Each successful session, every new milestone reached, deserves recognition. Treat yourself to a small reward, indulge in self-reflection, or share your triumph with your supportive community. Recognizing your efforts reinforces the positive association with Wall Pilates, keeping your motivation alive.

5. Keep It Varied and Fun:
Inject variety into your Wall Pilates routine to stave off monotony. Experiment with different exercises, explore various sequences and introduce music into your sessions. Making your workouts enjoyable transforms them from tasks into engaging experiences, ensuring you look forward to each session.

6. Prioritize Consistency Over Intensity:
Consistency is the bedrock of success in Wall Pilates. Establish a constant routine that fits seamlessly into your lifestyle. While intensity is essential, prioritize regularity. Even shorter, consistent sessions can yield remarkable results over time. The commitment to regular practice forms the backbone of your journey.

7. Visualize Your Progress:
Create a visual (and personal) representation of your progress and goals. Whether it's a vision board with images that embody your fitness aspirations or a chart showcasing your evolving abilities, visual aids can be powerful motivators. They serve as constant reminders of the transformative journey you're on.

Remember that motivation is dynamic as you integrate these practical strategies into your Wall Pilates routine. It requires nurturing, adaptation, and the occasional recalibration. Embrace the process, celebrate your commitment, and let the journey of Wall Pilates be a physical endeavor and a holistic, uplifting experience.

Elevating Your Routine and Fostering Long-Term Commitment

Embarking on the transformative journey of Wall Pilates isn't just about the exercises; it's about seamlessly weaving this enriching practice into your daily life. Here's a guide that not only helps you overcome common barriers but also nurtures a lasting commitment to your well-being:

Embrace Daily Integration:
Make Wall Pilates an integral part of your daily routine by carving out dedicated time slots. Recognize that even brief, focused sessions can yield substantial benefits. Whether it's a morning stretch, a midday energy boost, or an evening wind-down, find pockets of time that align with your schedule.

Conquer Time and Space Constraints:
Limited time and space need not hinder your Wall Pilates journey. Opt for shorter, targeted sessions that suit your daily demands. Identify small spaces to unfold your mat and engage in transformative movements. Flexibility is the key – your practice adapts to your lifestyle.

Create a Ritual:
Establish a ritual around your Wall Pilates routine to signal the transition into your practice. Whether setting aside a specific time each day, creating a calming environment with soft lighting, or incorporating soothing music, rituals help anchor your practice in consistency.

Consistency Over Intensity:
Prioritize consistency over lengthy, intensive sessions. Even a few minutes each day foster habit formation and contribute significantly to your overall well-being. Consistency not only accelerates physical progress but also deepens the mental and emotional benefits of Wall Pilates.

Personal Growth Through Practice:
View your Wall Pilates journey as a catalyst for personal growth. As you commit to consistent practice, observe the evolution in physical abilities, mental resilience, and emotional well-being. The challenges overcome on the mat mirror the triumphs in your daily life, fostering a holistic sense of growth.

Set Realistic Goals:
Set reachable goals that align with your current lifestyle and fitness level. Whether it's mastering a new pose or progressing to more advanced sequences, realistic goals

maintain motivation. Celebrate each accomplishment, reinforcing the positive cycle of growth and commitment.

Integrate Mindful Practices:
Extend the principles of Wall Pilates beyond the mat by embracing mindful practices. Incorporate mindfulness into your daily routine – focus on your breath during routine tasks, practice body awareness, and carry the principles of balance and stability into your daily activities.

Make It Enjoyable:
Infuse joy into your Wall Pilates practice. Experiment with different exercises, explore creative sequences, and perhaps even enlist a workout buddy. The more enjoyable and tailored to your preferences your sessions become, the more sustainable and fulfilling your commitment will be.

Evolve with Your Practice:
Recognising personal growth is a dynamic journey. Let your Wall Pilates practice evolve organically. Modify exercises, explore variations, and adapt your routine as your strength and flexibility improve. Embracing evolution ensures that your commitment remains fresh and invigorating.

As you seamlessly integrate Wall Pilates into your daily routines and commit to the journey of personal growth, remember that each session is a step toward holistic well-being. By overcoming barriers and fostering consistency, you sculpt your body and nurture a lifelong commitment to your health and vitality.

Chapter 2: Setting the Stage for Success

Starting a Wall Pilates challenge is not just about the exercises; it involves creating an environment that fosters focus, consistency, and overall well-being. Here's a comprehensive guide to help you make the most of this transformative journey!

- <u>Choose a Dedicated Space:</u> Designate a specific area for your Wall Pilates practice. This enhances focus and creates a mental cue for the transition into your workout routine. Opt for a space with enough room to stretch your arms and legs comfortably. Clear away potential obstacles to ensure a safe and uninterrupted practice.
- <u>Play with Lighting:</u> Natural light can invigorate your practice, but if that's not feasible, opt for soft, diffused lighting. Avoid harsh, direct lights that might cause distraction.
- <u>Set the Ambiance:</u> Create a calming atmosphere with soothing colors, plants, or inspiring quotes. Tailor the ambiance to make your Pilates space an inviting haven.

Checklist for Wall Pilates

Essentials:

- Mat: Ensure a comfortable and non-slip surface.
- Sturdy Wall: Your support and resistance anchor.
- Comfortable Attire: Wear breathable and flexible clothing.

Optional Enhancements:

- Pilates Ball: Adds variety and challenge.
- Resistance Bands: Enhance strength training.
- Small Pillow or Cushion: Supports the lower back during specific exercises.

Household Alternatives:
Get creative with household items – a rolled-up towel or cushion as a makeshift Pilates ball or a sturdy chair for specific modifications. The key is adaptability.

Strategies for Readiness

<u>Establish a Routine:</u> Set a consistent time for your Wall Pilates challenge. Whether it's the tranquility of morning or evening decompression, a routine establishes a sense of commitment.

<u>Preliminary Stretching:</u> Begin with gentle stretches to awaken your muscles and improve flexibility. Focus on areas that will be engaged during your Pilates session. You can use the Warm-Up flows you can find inside Chapter 3!

<u>Stay Hydrated:</u> Vital to a successful workout. Ensure you're well-hydrated before and after your session to support endurance and recovery.

<u>Mindful Mental Preparation:</u> Take a few moments to center yourself mentally. Deep breaths, a brief meditation, or even a moment of pure gratitude can set a positive tone for your practice.

Mental and Physical Strategies

<u>Focus on Breath Work:</u> Center your attention on mindful breathing. The rhythmic flow of breath enhances each movement and promotes a mind-body connection. You can follow the breathing instructions associated with each position you will find from Chapter 3 onwards.

<u>Gradual Progression:</u> If you're new to Wall Pilates, start gradually. Familiarize yourself with the movements, gradually increasing intensity. Progression over perfection is the key.

<u>Listen to Your Body:</u> Pay attention to your body's cues. If an exercise feels uncomfortable or causes pain, modify or skip it. Your well-being takes precedence.

<u>Post-Challenge Reflection:</u> After each session, take a moment for reflection. Note your achievements, any challenges faced, and how you felt physically and mentally. This reflective practice enhances mindfulness and growth.
By following these comprehensive strategies, you'll optimize your Wall Pilates challenge and create an environment conducive to long-term well-being.
Remember, this journey is about cultivating a holistic commitment to your health and vitality.

Chapter 3: Safety Tips

Safety is paramount in your Wall Pilates journey as the foundation for a fulfilling and injury-free experience. Emphasizing the crucial impact of proper form and alignment during exercises is critical.

This includes being mindful of your body's signals and distinguishing between discomfort, a sign of muscle fatigue, and pain, which could indicate potential injury. Furthermore, advocating for a gradual increase in exercise difficulty helps prevent overexertion, ensuring you challenge yourself within safe limits. It's crucial to strike a balance with the wall – a valuable support but not an over-reliance that compromises correct form.

You lay the groundwork for a sustainable and health-focused fitness journey by approaching Wall Pilates with a safety-first mindset. Let's find out how!

Balance, Support, and Caution

Understanding how to leverage the wall for balance and support is fundamental in Wall Pilates. Detailed guidance on using the wall as a stabilizing force ensures proper execution of movements, enhancing both safety and effectiveness.

However, caution must be exercised against excessive reliance on the wall, as this can lead to incorrect form and diminished engagement of targeted muscle groups. Striking a balance, where the wall provides support without becoming a crutch, is imperative. This nuanced approach maximizes the benefits of Wall Pilates while focusing on each exercise's safety and integrity. We will discover together how to perform each position safely and easily.

The Pace of Progression: Gradual and Controlled

As we saw earlier, encouraging a gradual increase in exercise difficulty forms the linchpin of a safe and sustainable Wall Pilates routine.
Rushing into advanced movements can invite overexertion and increase the risk of injury. Instead, advocate for a step-by-step progression that aligns with your fitness level.

Similarly, highlighting the value of a slow and controlled pace in executing movements underscores the importance of mindfulness. By moving deliberately and with control, you enhance the effectiveness of each exercise and minimize the likelihood of strain or injury, fostering a safer and more rewarding fitness journey. I will help you with that within the following chapters and routines!

Tailored Warm-Up Techniques for Wall Pilates

Before delving into the stimulating world of Wall Pilates, ensuring your body is primed and ready is paramount.

Explore a range of warm-up exercises meticulously designed to complement the unique demands of Wall Pilates. These targeted warm-up techniques aim to awaken key muscle groups, enhance flexibility, and prepare your body and mind for the following enriching movements.

Incorporating these purposeful warm-up exercises into your routine will pave the way for a more effective and injury-resistant Wall Pilates experience.

Here's the deal with Wall Pilates—it's all about those slow movements, making it perfect for beginners and seniors. It's an excellent warm-up before you dive into your regular workout routine.

Take it easy and confidently do these exercises right before your daily workout. Rock some comfy, stretchy, and breathable clothes—organic fabric, if possible. And, of course, sip on a glass of water before you kick things off.

Let's dive into these poses (and keep reading for how long to hold each one).

Warm Up Exercises

1. Wall Roll and Stretch

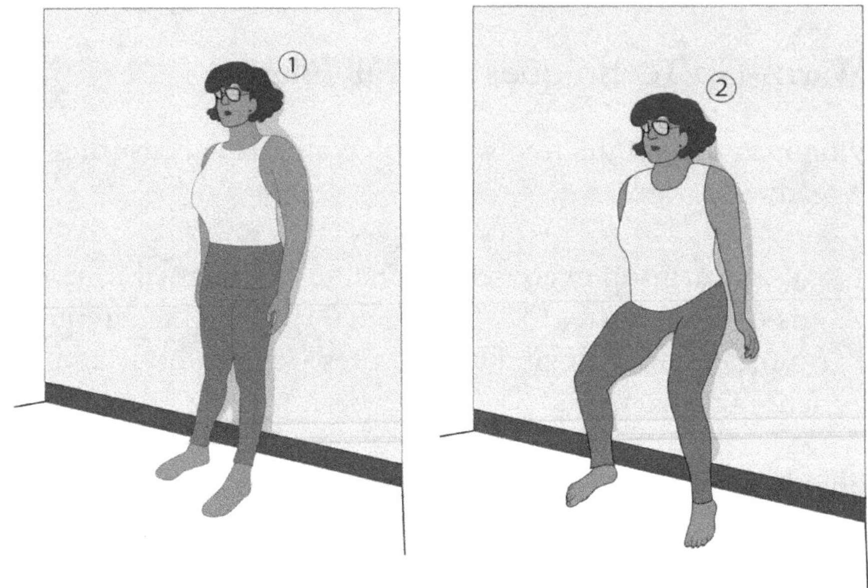

- Stand tall against the wall, back snug against it.
- Step your feet away from the wall about six inches, tighten that core, and let your shoulders chill.
- Inhale as you slowly roll down the wall, inch by inch. Feel those back muscles stretch on the way down.
- Exhale when you reach the bottom, arms hanging out by your sides. Hold it for a couple of breaths.
- Inhale and gently push yourself back up, then repeat about five times.

Body Awareness Tips: Stay mindful of your body as you gradually roll down the wall, paying attention to each part of your spine. This will help maximize the stretch in your back muscles.

Breath Tips: Coordinate your breath with the movement, inhaling as you descend and exhaling at the bottom, enhancing the flow and mindfulness of the exercise.

Safety Tips: Ensure safety by maintaining proper core engagement and avoiding overextension, allowing for controlled movement.

Body Parts Engaged: Upper body, lower body, back (spine, dorsals), core (abdominals).

2. Hip-Opener Leverage

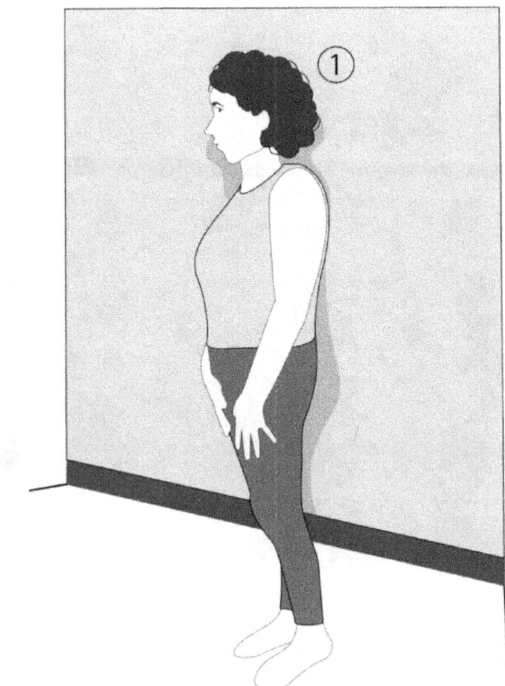 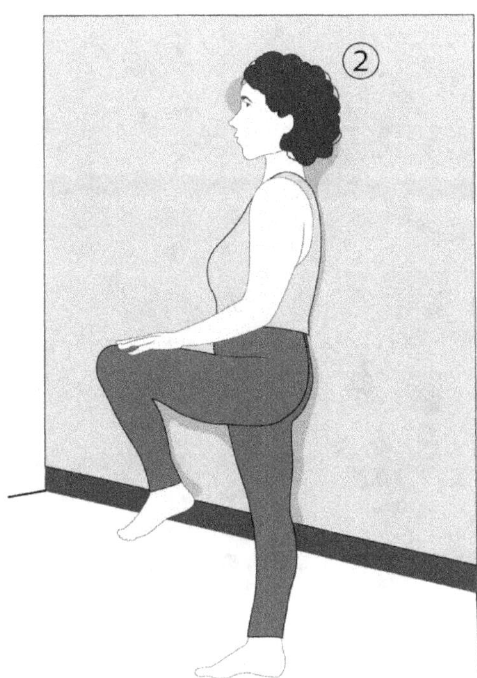

- Stand beside the wall with one hand resting on it.
- Lift one leg to the side, ensuring your thigh is parallel to the floor. Keep your hips level and facing forward. Drop your inner hand on your raised thigh for support.
- Exhale as you press the leg into your hand, opening it to the side.
- Hold the pose for a couple of breaths.
- Inhale, release the leg and switch to the other side.

Body Awareness Tips: Keeping your hips level and facing forward while opening your leg to the side, ensuring proper alignment and engagement.

Breath Tips: Sync your breath with the movement, exhaling as you press the leg into your hand and inhaling as you release, promoting relaxation and control.

Safety Tips: Prioritize safety by using the wall for support, preventing overreaching, and ensuring stability throughout the hip-opening exercise.

Body Parts Engaged: Upper body, lower body, hips (abductors), core (abdominals).

3. Swing and Stretch

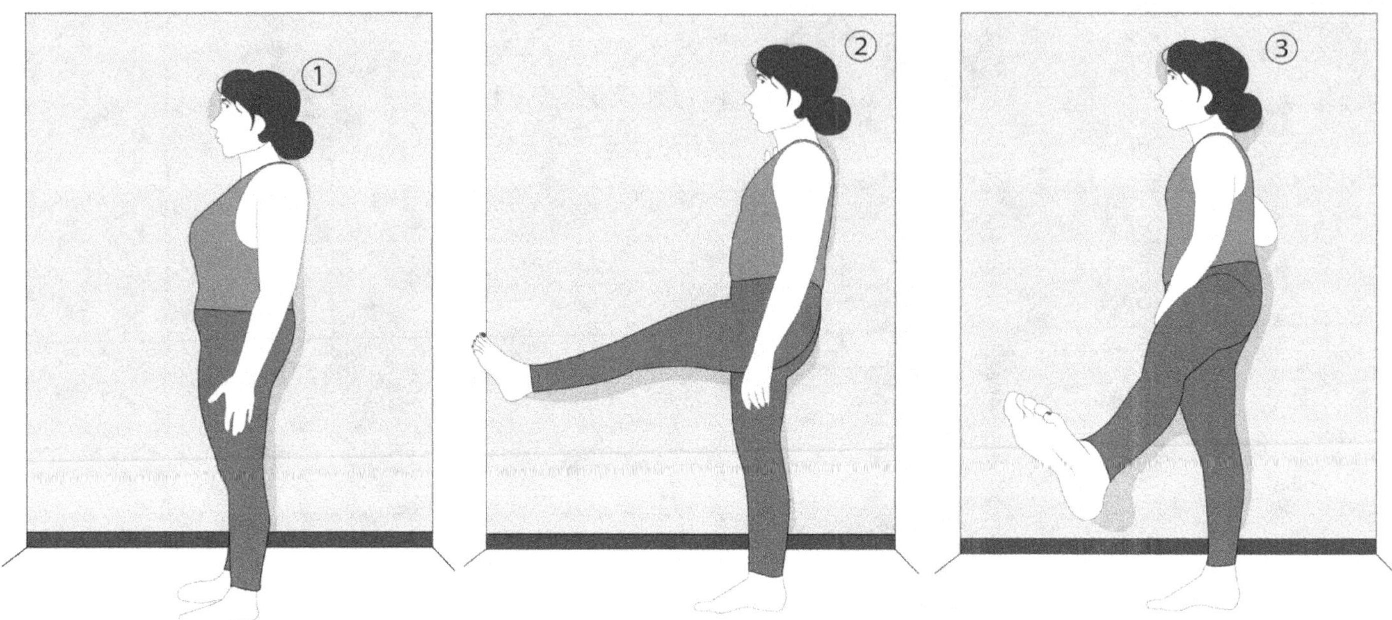

- Stand next to your wall with one hand for support.
- Lift your outer leg, aiming for a parallel thigh-to-floor situation. Keep that hips level and facing forward.
- Swing your leg out to the side, reaching for the stars.
- Bring it back to the starting position with style.
- Repeat the leg-swinging fun on the other side.

Body Awareness Tips: Heighten body awareness by maintaining level hips and controlled leg swing, feeling the stretch and strengthening effects throughout the movement.

Breath Tips: Breathe rhythmically during the leg swing, inhaling as you raise the leg and exhaling as you bring it back to the starting position, fostering a smooth and controlled motion.

Safety Tips: Exercise caution by focusing on controlled movements, avoiding excessive swinging, and using the wall for support to prevent losing balance.

Body Parts Engaged: Upper body, lower body, legs (abductors, adductors), core (abdominals).

4. Active Calf Release

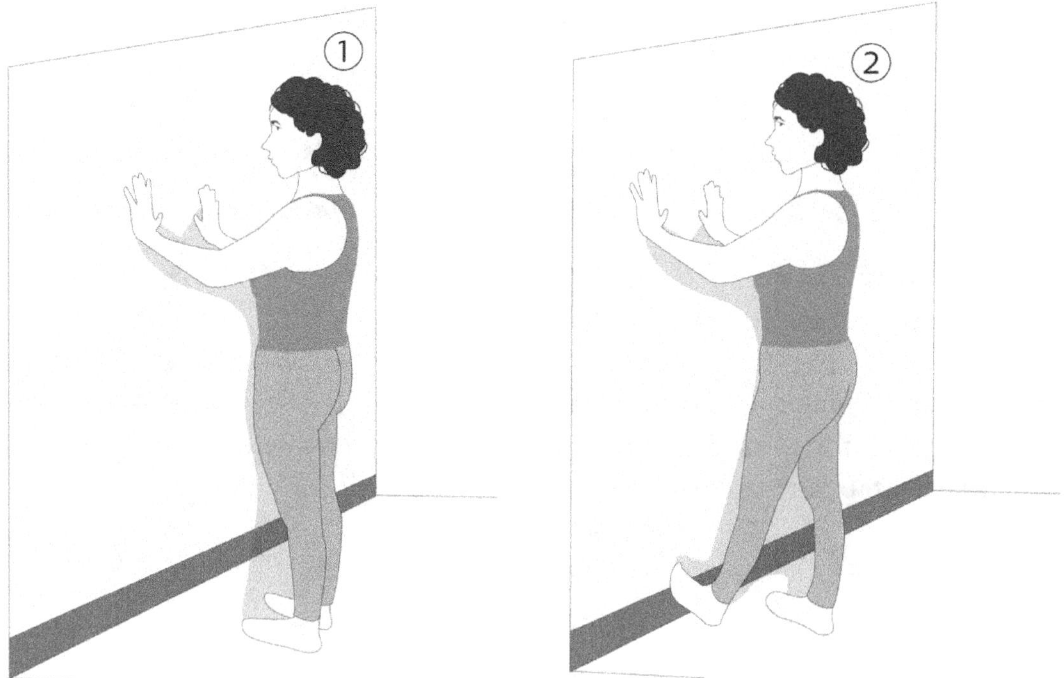

- Hang out next to the wall again, palms casually on it at shoulder height. Step the right leg back about 40 inches, keeping that heel on the floor.
- Now, with your left leg extended, place your toes on the wall, while placing your heel on the ground 15-20 inches apart.
- In practice, you will find yourself with both legs extended, only the right one further back and with the heel on the ground, while the left one is closer to the wall and with the toes resting on the wall and the heel on the ground.
- Feel that pleasant stretch in the left calf and all over your left leg. Hold it for a couple of breaths. Release and switch to the other side.

Body Awareness Tips: Ensure proper form as you lean against the wall for an active calf stretch, experiencing the release in the targeted muscles.

Breath Tips: Practice deep, intentional breaths during the calf stretch, aiding in relaxation and allowing for a more effective release of tension in the muscles.

Safety Tips: Prioritize safety by keeping the heel on the floor during the calf stretch, preventing strain and ensuring a safe and effective muscle stretch.

Body Parts Engaged: Lower body, calves, and quadriceps.

Post-Workout Rituals: Cooling Down and Stretching

The journey doesn't conclude with the final Wall Pilates movement; it extends to the post-workout phase. Stressing the importance of a proper cool-down and stretching routine after each session is integral to aiding recovery and preventing muscle stiffness. Dedicating time to these post-workout rituals enhances flexibility, reduces muscle tension, and improves overall well-being.

Emphasize the holistic approach to fitness — it's not just about the exertion; it's also about the care you extend to your body afterward.

Turn your Wall Pilates session into a perfect cooldown after your workout. Here's a pro tip: perform these exercises calmly and confidently after daily training. Hold each pose for the established time (keep reading).

Cool Down Exercises

1. Seated Opposing Toe-Tapping

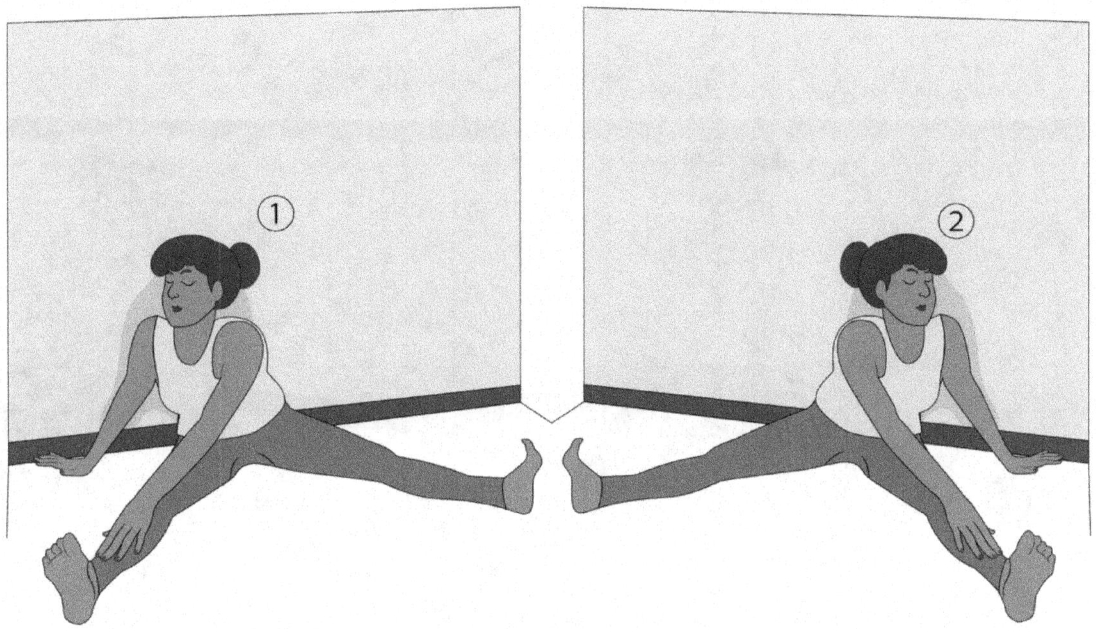

- Sit on the floor with your back against the wall, legs stretched out.
- Gently spread your legs hip-width apart. Squeeze your abs, pressing your back into the wall.
- Reach out the toes of your right foot with your left hand, then switch to left foot and right hand.
- Be mindful on alternating sides for 45 seconds or as long as needed.

Body Awareness Tips: Foster body awareness by maintaining a robust seated position against the wall, focusing on core engagement and controlled leg movements during the toe-tapping exercise.

Breath Tips: Coordinate your breath with the tapping motion, exhaling as you reach for your toes and inhaling as you return to the starting position, promoting a rhythmic and mindful practice.

Safety Tips: Ensure safety by avoiding overextension and tapping gently, respecting your body's limits to prevent strain or discomfort.

Body Parts Engaged: Lower body, core (abdominals, obliques), legs (quadriceps, hamstrings).

2. Seated Spinal Twist

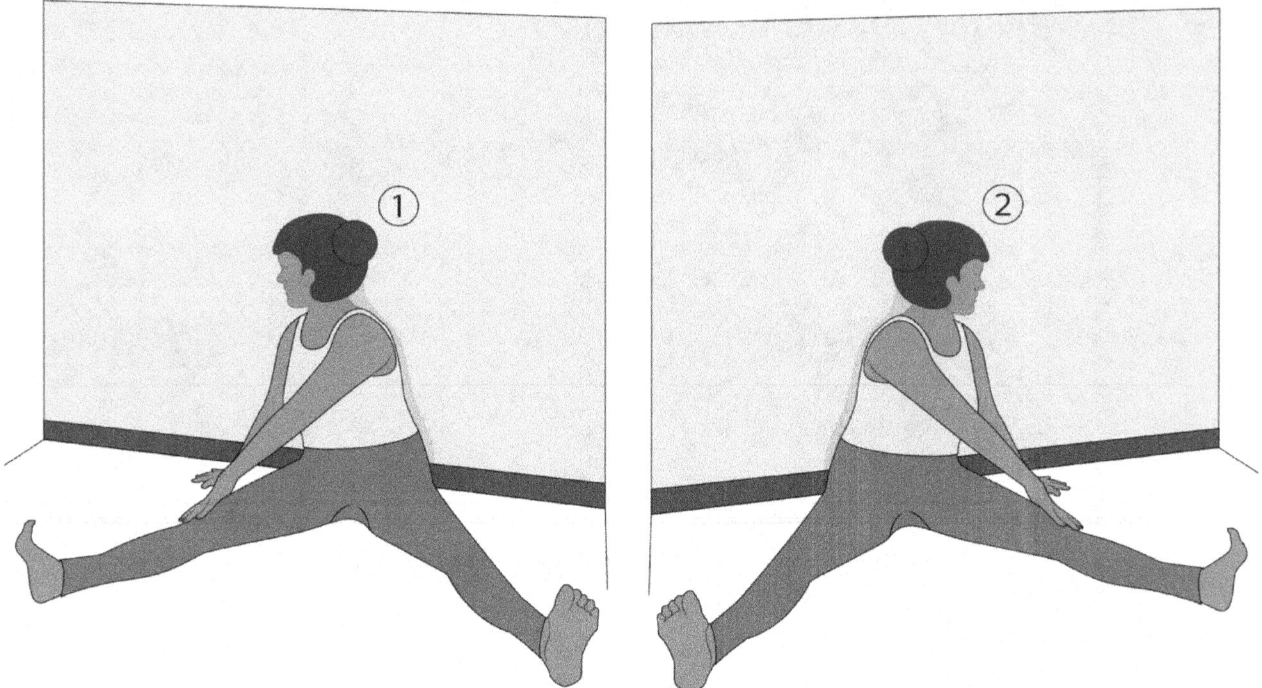

*   Sit on the floor with your back against the wall, legs extended.
*   Spread your legs hip-width apart and tighten your abs.
*   Rotate your torso to the right, reaching out with your left hand to the right knee. Reverse the twist, reaching out with your right hand to the left knee.
*   Be mindful on alternating sides for 45 seconds or as long as needed.

Body Awareness Tips: Cultivate body awareness by sitting against the wall with proper alignment, engaging your abs, and rotating your torso smoothly during the spinal twist.

Breath Tips: Sync your breath with the twisting movement, exhaling as you twist to each side and inhaling as you return to the center, enhancing the flow and relaxation of the stretch.

Safety Tips: Exercise caution by avoiding excessive twisting, listening to your body's signals, and adapting the range of motion to your comfort level.

Body Parts Engaged: Lower body, core (abdominals, obliques), spine (thoracic and lumbar regions).

3. Butterfly Stretch

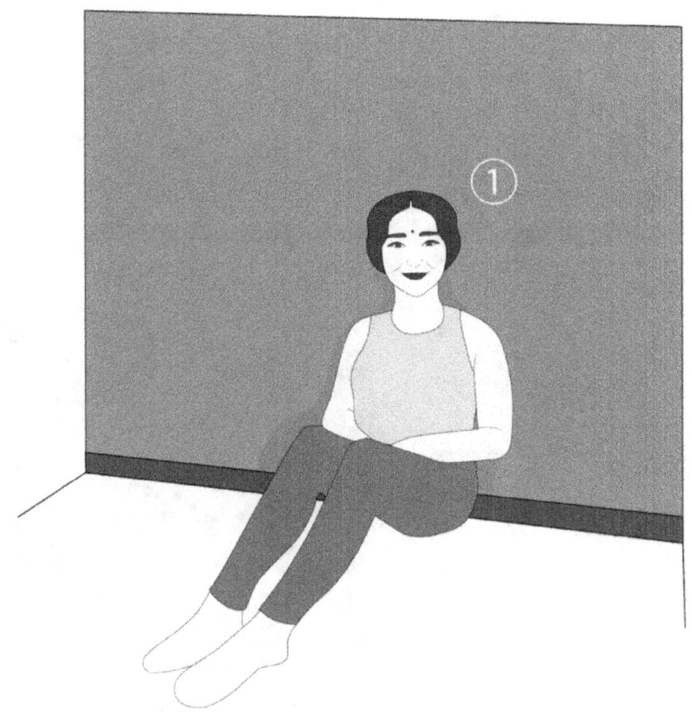
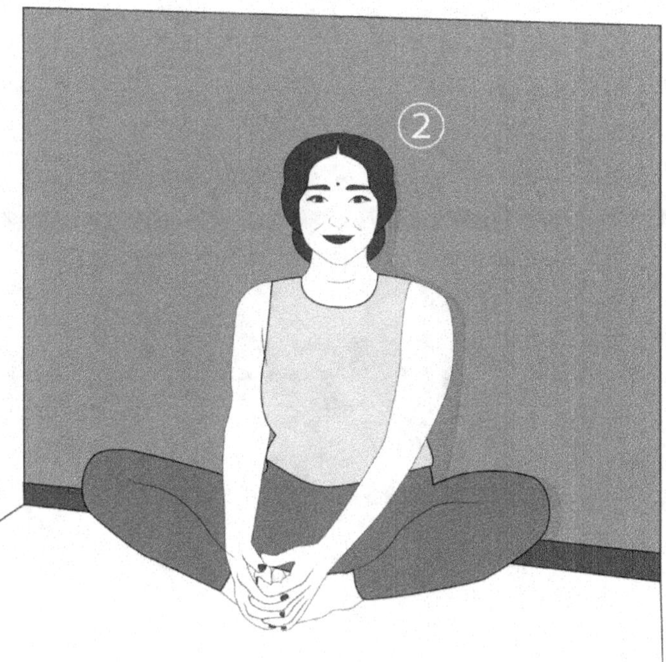

- Sit against the wall with your legs bent and the soles of your feet touching.
- Let your knees open to the sides and press your back into the wall.
- Then, trying to keep your back straight, bring your chest towards your heels but without forcing the movement.
- Hold for a couple of breaths and relax.

Body Awareness Tips: Heighten body awareness by sitting against the wall with the soles of your feet touching, focusing on the gentle opening of your knees during the butterfly stretch.

Breath Tips: Practice deep breaths during the stretch, promoting a sense of release and relaxation.

Safety Tips: Prioritize safety by avoiding forceful stretching, allowing your knees to open naturally, and using the wall for support to maintain proper alignment.

Body Parts Engaged: Lower body, hips (adductors), inner thighs, core (abdominals)

4. Seated Forward Bend

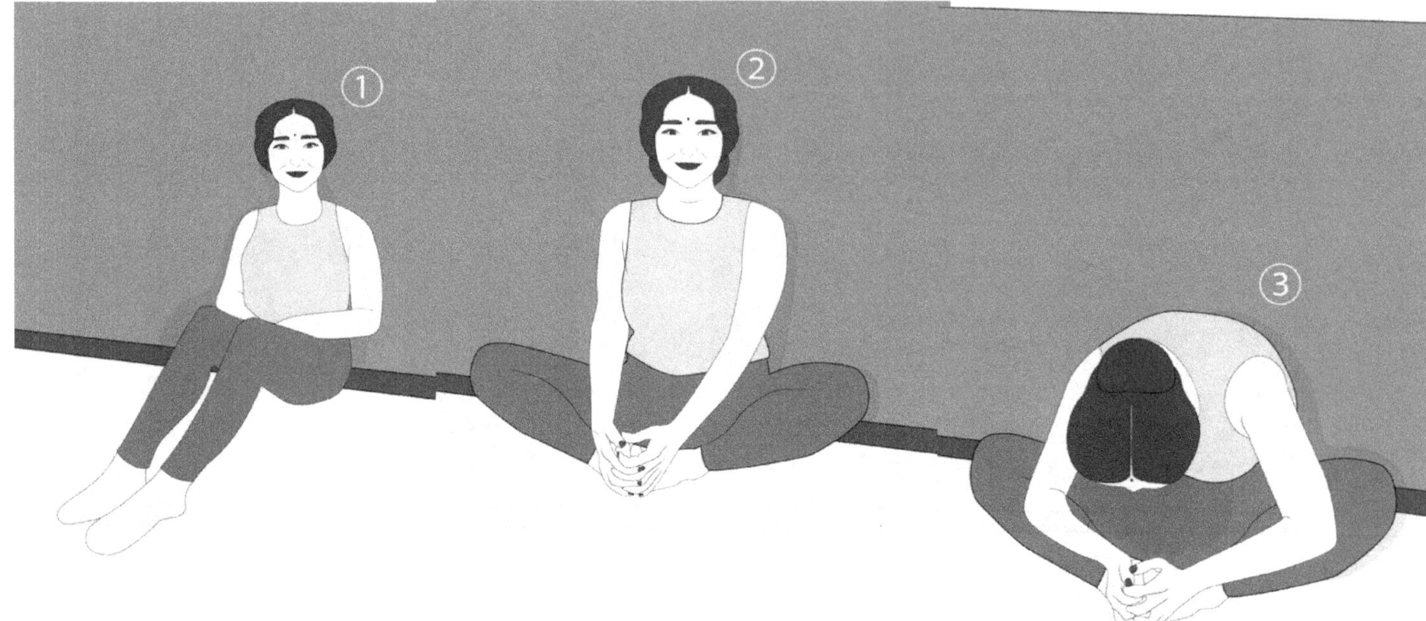

- Sit against the wall with your legs bent and the soles of your feet touching, as in the previous position.
- Let your knees open to the sides, pressing your back into the wall.
- Now, lean forward from the hips, and let your head and shoulders hang down.
- Hold for a couple of breaths and return to the starting position.
- Enjoy this relaxing cooldown routine, and let your wall support you in unwinding after your workout!

Body Awareness Tips: Stay attuned to your body by sitting against the wall, opening your knees, and reaching forward from the hips during the forward bend, feeling the stretch along your back.

Breath Tips: Breathe deeply during the forward bend and inhale to lengthen your spine; then, exhale to deepen the stretch, enhancing the therapeutic effects of the pose.

Safety Tips: Exercise caution by avoiding overreaching, allowing a gradual stretch, and using the wall for support to prevent strain during the forward bend.

Body Parts Engaged: Lower body, back (spine), hamstrings, core (abdominals).

Recognizing the Need for Rest

Knowing when to rest is a skill that enhances the safety and sustainability of your Wall Pilates practice. Understanding the signs that indicate the need for a break or a lighter workout day is essential. This might include persistent fatigue, muscle soreness beyond the usual, or any discomfort that feels more than the typical post-exercise sensations. Acknowledging these signals and giving your body the rest it requires is a proactive measure to prevent burnout and potential injuries, fostering a healthier and more balanced fitness routine.

What to do in these circumstances? Rest! If you notice that your muscles are still struggling to recover after an intense workout, give them rest and sustenance, perhaps alternating Wall Pilates with a run or walk.

You can also opt for alternating the various muscle groups (our 28-day plan is built based on this principle) or a shorter workout (e.g., 5-10 minutes).

Knowing When to Stop

The concept of distinguishing between good pain, such as muscle fatigue that accompanies a productive workout, and bad pain, indicative of potential injury, serves as a fundamental guide, even in Wall Pilates.

Recognizing these distinctions allows you to tailor your exercises to your body's current capacity, ensuring a challenging yet safe routine. It's crucial to listen to the signals of your body, understand when discomfort surpasses the expected fatigue, and know when to stop what you are doing.

Basically, if you encounter any sharp pain or undue strain, it's a clear sign to halt the exercise and give your body the rest it needs. Put simply, if you ever feel a sudden, intense pain or an unusual level of strain during an exercise, it's crucial to stop that specific movement immediately. This discomfort could be a sign that your body is being pushed too hard or that there might be a risk of injury. Taking a break allows your muscles and joints to recover and prevents potential harm. Listen to your body's signals, and if something doesn't feel right, it's better to pause and reassess rather than push through and risk injury. It's all about prioritizing your well-being and ensuring a safe and effective workout experience.

Safety Recap: Reiterating the 'Safety First' Mindset

Summarizing all safety tips discussed, this recap reminds you of the fundamental principles governing your practice for making it great and safe. By prioritizing safety at every step – from form and balance to gradual progression and post-workout care- you solidify a fitness foundation that transforms your body with longevity and well-being in mind. Here it is!

- Understand how to use the wall for balance and support, enhancing safety and effectiveness.
- Caution against excessive reliance on the wall to maintain form and engage muscle groups effectively. Strive for a balance that maximizes benefits without compromising exercise integrity.
- Prioritize a primed and ready body before diving into Wall Pilates.
- Explore warm-up exercises designed for Wall Pilates, awakening muscles and enhancing flexibility to ensure a practical and injury-resistant experience.
- Master utilizing the wall for stability understanding its role during exercises.
- Advocate for gradually increasing exercise difficulty for a safe and sustainable Wall Pilates routine.
- Emphasize a slow and controlled pace in executing movements, fostering mindfulness and minimizing the risk of strain or injury.
- Enhance flexibility, reduce muscle tension, and contribute to overall well-being by dedicating time to post-workout care.
- Acknowledge signs of persistent fatigue, unusual muscle soreness, or discomfort beyond typical post-exercise sensations for a proactive and balanced fitness routine.
- Develop the skill of recognizing signals that indicate the need for rest or a lighter workout day.
- Prioritize safety at every step, from form and balance to gradual progression and post-workout care, for a fitness foundation prioritizing longevity and well-being.

Chapter 4: Unraveling the Essence of Pilates Breathing

Have you ever questioned if there's a correct way to breathe? Pilates answers this query by emphasizing the profound impact of proper breathing on your workout and well-being. In this chapter, we dive into Pilates breathing, where every inhalation and exhalation transforms into a strengthening exercise, exceeding the boundaries of conventional respiration.

The roots of Pilates' breathing are linked to Joseph Pilates, who, in his 1960 book, underscores the vitality of correct breathing. Pilates points out how lazy breathing can adversely affect your body, making your lungs a haven for harmful germs. Pilates breathing extends beyond mere inhaling and exhaling; it's a holistic approach that optimizes lung function by engaging core muscles.

Also, a well-executed breathing technique should induce post-workout relaxation, gradually acclimating your body to changes in pace, calming muscles, and freeing your mind from physical fatigue. The ideal breath is smooth, steady, and controlled, fostering a sense of balance and calmness.

In addition, learning to breathe carefully during the positions and when transitioning between positions helps you perform the exercises correctly and better, increasing flexibility, concentration, and joy.

Last but not least, Pilates offers a unique approach to breathing in contrast to many other exercise routines. There's no strict prescription for inhaling or exhaling in a predetermined manner or at specific intervals. Instead, in Pilates, we emphasize aligning the rhythm and strength of your breath with the nature of the exercise at hand. For instance, adopting a calm and natural breathing pattern is encouraged during restorative movements. Conversely, a more robust and vigorous breathing style is recommended for more dynamic exercises, such as the hundred, to complement the heightened activity.

Unlocking the Power of Pilates Breathing

Pilates breathing stands apart from the conventional techniques taught in aerobics or weightlifting. It's a specialized method designed to enhance your breathing effectively while strengthening your diaphragm and core muscles.

1. Energize Your Body
Beyond being a mere proof of life, breathing is the engine that continuously supplies energy to your cells, including muscle cells. Let's simplify the science: breathing is like the energy source for your body cells, especially your muscles. Your muscles need a fuel called adenosine triphosphate (ATP) to do their job. ATP is made when your body mixes glucose (a type of sugar) with oxygen from the air you breathe. So, when you breathe, you're basically helping your muscles get the energy they need to move.

2. Cleanses Your Body
Breathing is a natural detoxifying process, generating energy while producing CO2 as a byproduct. Naturally, your body aims to eliminate this toxic compound. Resounding exhales echo Joseph Pilates' wisdom to "squeeze every atom from your lungs" to cleanse your body of CO2 and re-oxygenate. This prepares your lungs to welcome ample oxygen, revitalizing and rejuvenating your entire being.

3. Calms Your Mind And Reduces Stress
Conscious breathing during Pilates workouts transforms it into a meditative practice. Scientifically proven to relieve stress[8], a dedicated Pilates practice promises physical benefits, emotional tranquility, and mental clarity.

4. Core Engagement
Pilates breathing isn't just about oxygenating your body; it actively involves your core. As you practice specialized breathing techniques, your diaphragm and surrounding core muscles are actively engaged. This intentional involvement enhances the strength and stability of your core, contributing to improved posture, balance, and overall functional fitness. So, beyond the physical and mental benefits, Pilates breathing becomes a dynamic core workout, fortifying your body from the inside out.

Why is it important to breathe correctly in Pilates?

Understanding the significance of proper breathing in Pilates is crucial. Your breath has the power to influence your exercise experience significantly.
Therefore, to maximize the benefits of your Pilates routines, it's essential to grasp the art of breathing in Pilates. Continue reading to discover how :)

---

[8] https://hbr.org/2020/09/research-why-breathing-is-so-effective-at-reducing-stress

Pilates Breathing Techniques

1. Diaphragmatic Breathing

In Pilates, our attention is directed toward critical muscles associated with breathing, namely the diaphragm and oblique muscles. The diaphragm is pivotal as it serves as a division between the abdominal and thoracic cavities.

During inhalation, the diaphragm contracts, prompting the intake of air and causing a subtle rise in the abdomen. If an individual predominantly engages the diaphragm for breathing, neglecting the involvement of intercostal and other muscles, the result may be significant abdominal protrusion upon each inhalation instead of the intended expansion of the ribcage.

Also known as deep-belly breathing, this technique involves fully engaging your diaphragm during inhalation.

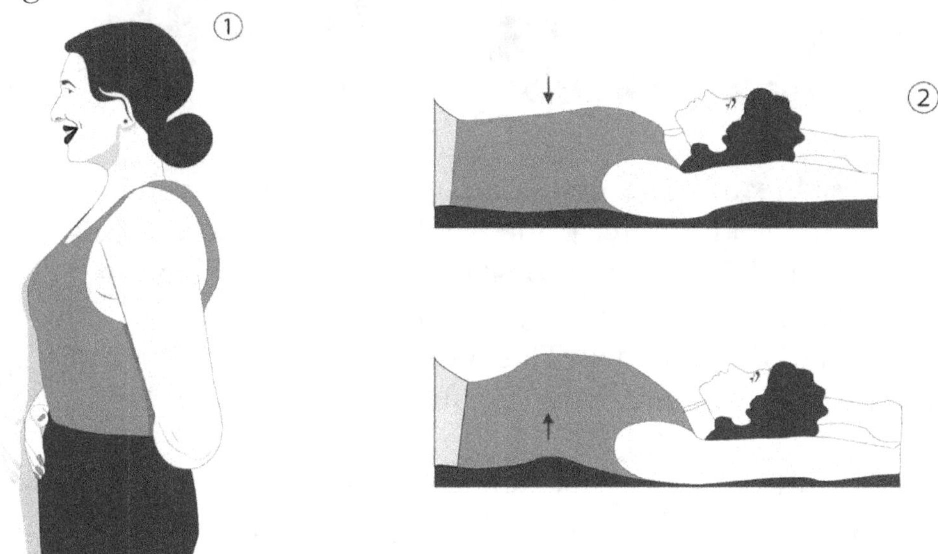

Here's how:
- Find a comfortable position, whether standing or lying on your back.
- Release tension on neck and shoulders.
- If you stand, place one hand on your belly and the other one on the back (as in pose 1).
- If you lie on your back, raise your arms above the head (pose 2).
- Inhale deeply, trying the sensation of the air enter your nostrils and focusing on your abdomen rising while keeping your chest still.
- Exhale slowly through your lips, tightening your stomach and allowing your belly to return to its original position.
- Repeat ten times or practice for 3-5 minutes.

2. Lateral Breathing

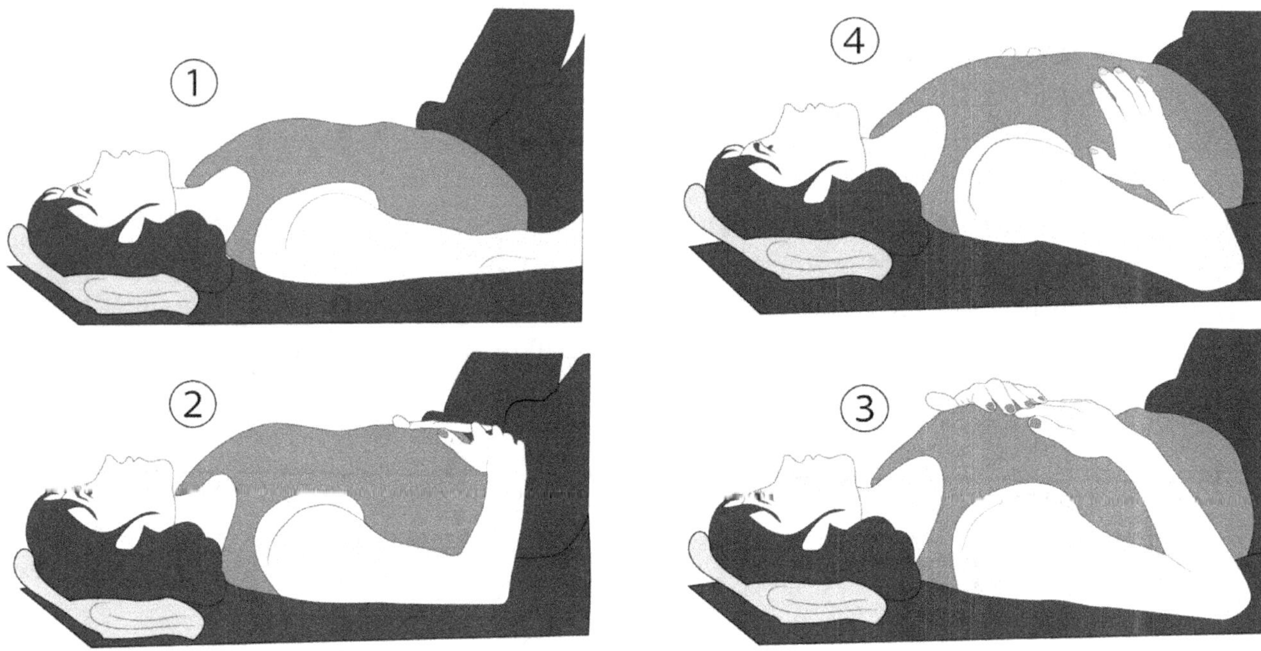

Learning lateral breathing becomes crucial as it teaches the optimal way of breathing, the ribcage to move in all three planes while the abdomen expands slightly. In Wall Pilates, we call this "three-dimensional breathing": we breathe laterally into the flanks (lateral rib arches), backward and forward into the rib arch. Also, the breathing flows somewhat toward the abdomen. This breathing method can enhance spinal mobility, alleviate stress, and promote better digestion.

Optimal breathing occurs in three dimensions, involving expansion forward and back, sideways, and upward and downward movements in the body. Unfortunately, many people are accustomed to shallow breathing, primarily in the chest, with tucked-in stomachs, leading to tension and restricted movement.

Why lateral breathing? It engages your core, stabilizing your trunk and providing extra support to your spine during workouts. As you master this technique, enhanced performance and results await you after every Pilates session.

Here is the how-to progression:

- Lie on your back with bent knees. Keep your shoulders relaxed and away from your ears, maintaining a neutral spine position with all-natural spinal curves.
- To understand how the flow of air moves three-dimensionally inside the rib cage, we take 3-4 natural breaths with our arms extended along the body **(1)**.
- Then, take another 3-4 complete breaths (inhalation and exhalation) with hands positioned on the belly **(2)** and another 3-4 breaths (inhalation and exhalation) with your hands resting on your chest **(3)**.
- Remember to inhale through your nose, allowing air to fill your chest and ribs to expand in all directions. Relax your stomach, letting the lower belly expand slightly.
- Exhale through an open mouth, allowing ribs to return inwards towards your spine without force. Also, ensure your shoulders stay relaxed and don't rise during inhalation; they should remain down.
- Choosing one of your favorite hand positions, now inhale evenly through the entire ribcage, sending the air to all directions, maintaining length through the top of your head and a stable spine position.
- Experiment by putting both hands, respectively, on your right and left ribs to feel direct lateral movement during breathing **(4)**.
- Practice exhaling with an open mouth and a relaxed throat to prevent tension and facilitate better movement. Sighing the air out can be beneficial.
- Repeat this breathing exercise 3 times in all directions.

3. Bellows Breathing

This breath exercise heightens alertness and clears the mind, providing a sense of grounding. Additionally, it proves beneficial for digestion and metabolism enhancement. This is how to perform this exercise:

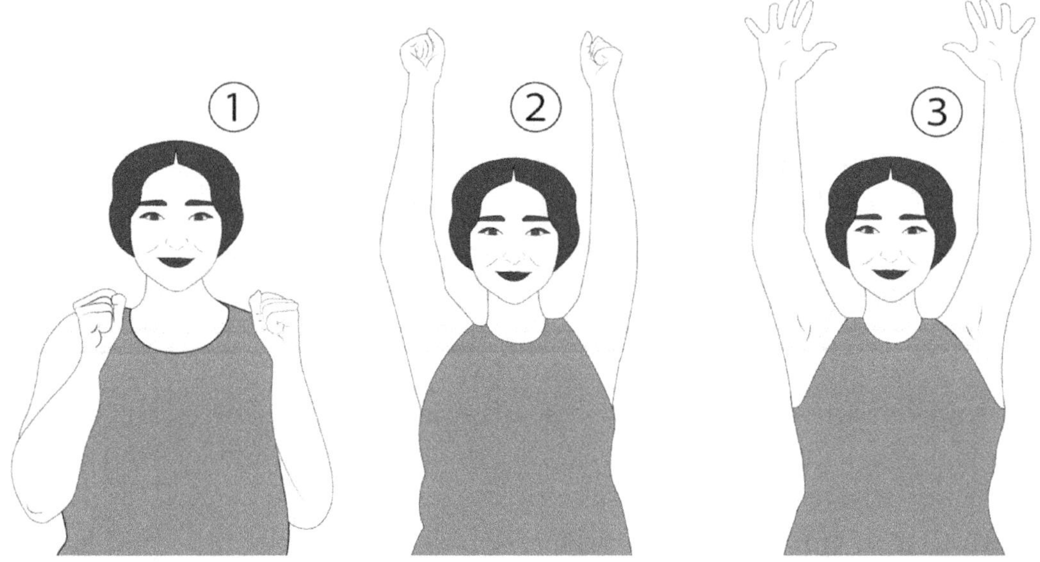

- Start standing with your back straight and your chin parallel to the floor, with your bent elbows, hands at shoulder height, and closed fists, palms facing each other (pose 1).
- Inhale through your nose, extend your arms overhead (pose 2), open your hands, and stretch your fingers wide (pose 3).
- Exhale forcefully through the nose as you lower your arms back to the starting position with closed fists at shoulder height.
- Repeat this sequence ten times, then relax and breathe normally.
- You can also perform this breathing technique while sitting.

Avoid practicing bellows breath if pregnant, menstruating, or dealing with conditions like high blood pressure, heart disease, epilepsy, vertigo, or recent abdominal surgery. Also, refrain from this form of breathing on a full stomach.

4. Box Breathing

Another relaxing breath exercise designed to calm the nervous system. This technique reduces stress hormone production, such as cortisol, and enhances stress response. Additionally, it improves focus, concentration, and lung capacity and aids detoxification by releasing toxins. How to perform Box Breathing:

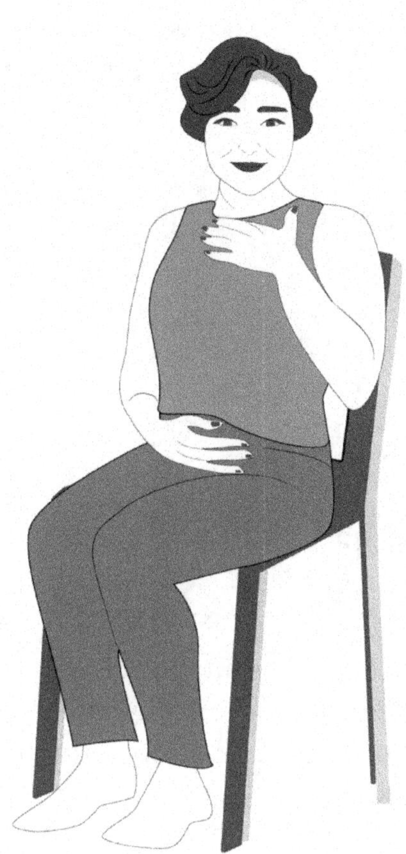

- You can stand or sit.

- Place one hand on your belly, and the other can touch your heart.

- Inhale slowly through the nostrils to the count of four to sense the belly (abdominal) expansion.

- Hold the inhale for a count of four.

- Exhale through the mouth for a count of four to feel the belly deflate.

- Hold the exhale again for a count of four.

- Repeat for several minutes as long as it starts feeling comfortable.

Potential Pitfalls in Pilates Breathing

There is a risk of breathing too forcefully, where the thoracic spine hyperextends during inhalation, and excessive tightness occurs in the abdominal wall during exhalation.
This should be actively avoided because, as previously highlighted, it alters the spine's alignment.

Another issue may arise when excessive inflation of the cheeks and overly compressed lips occur during exhalation, leading to tension in the neck and jaw muscles.

In order to avoid these risks, here is what you can do:

- Maintain a natural posture throughout the breathing process;

- Avoid excessive force in breathing;

- Keep facial muscles as relaxed as possible;

- Steer clear of intense abdominal retraction—activating the abdominal wall gently is critical.

Is Pilates breathing the exclusive correct method?

Definitely not! In essence, breathing techniques are not confined to right or wrong; instead, the crucial question revolves around the intended outcome of the breathing technique. Practices like Qi Gong, Yoga, and Tai Chi, among others, present diverse breathing methods, each exerting a unique impact on the body. In Pilates, the focus lies on fortifying the core and refining movement quality.

Post a Pilates session, we often recommend a brief breathing session. Transitioning from one breathing technique to another, day by day, provides a soothing mental effect, alleviating workout-induced tension. Additionally, this meditation fosters muscle recovery.

Breathing Mistakes and How to Correct Them

Identify common breathing errors frequently made by beginners, such as shallow breathing or holding the breath during some hard positions. To correct these mistakes, consider the following tips and exercises:

- Shallow Breathing Correction: Encourage deeper breaths by focusing on expanding your lungs fully. Practice diaphragmatic breathing, allowing your abdomen to rise and fall with each breath.

- Breath-Holding Correction: Develop awareness of breath-holding tendencies. Concentrate on maintaining a steady flow of breath during exercises. Incorporate a rhythmic count to ensure continuous inhalation and exhalation.

- Improved Breathing: Emphasize the importance of continuous, controlled breathing. Remind beginners to avoid abrupt inhalations or exhalations. Suggest a smooth, steady breath to enhance overall movement and coordination.

Enhancing Pilates Practice through Mindful Breathing

Follow the upcoming steps to incorporate mindfulness into your breathing routine:

Conscious Awareness:
Cultivate awareness of your breath as you move through Pilates exercises. Focus on the physical sensations of each inhale and exhale, bringing attention to the present moment.

Sync Breath with Movement:
Coordinate your breath with specific movements. Follow the instructions you find in this book for each of the positions you encounter, but as you become more expert at understanding your sensations, remember that the best way to match the breath to the position is to inhale during preparatory phases and exhale during exertion. This synchronization fosters a harmonious and natural connection between breath and body movement.

Mind-Body Connection:
Recognize the interconnectedness of breath and movement. Allow your breath to guide the flow of each exercise, promoting a more fluid and controlled Pilates practice.

Addressing common breathing mistakes and embracing mindful breathing techniques can optimize your Wall Pilates experience, promoting better coordination, concentration, and overall well-being.

Chapter 5: Core Stretches for Beginners

In this Chapter, we'll explore fundamental core stretches tailored for beginners using the support of a wall.

Whether you're new to Pilates or looking to refine your practice, these exercises aim to enhance your core strength, body awareness, and overall well-being.

Join us as we build the foundations for a fulfilling Pilates experience, bringing balance and vitality to your body through accessible and effective wall-assisted stretches.

Let's embark on this empowering exploration of Wall Pilates together!

1. Wall Push-Up to Plank

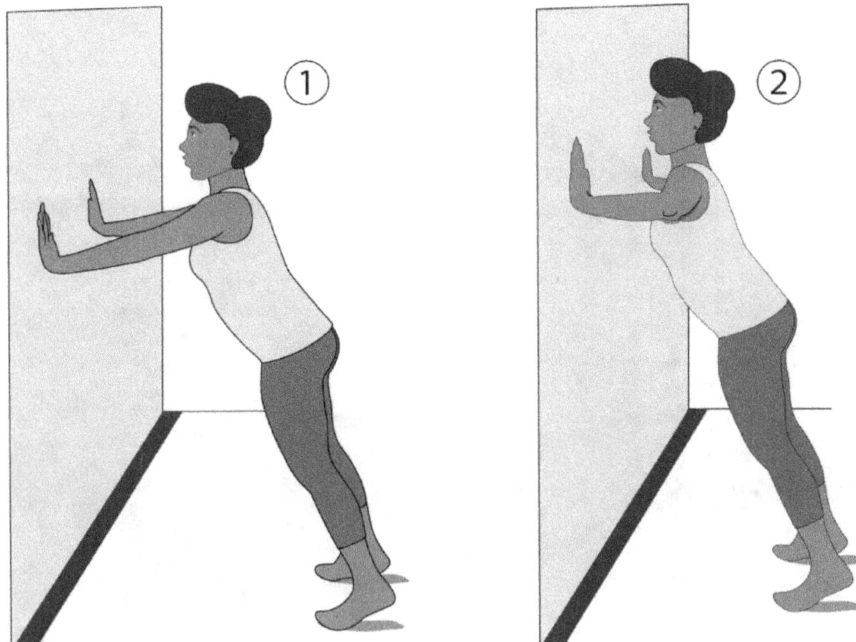

- Begin by standing in front of the wall, positioning your hands a little bit wider than shoulder-width apart, pressed against the surface.

- Activate your core muscles and take a step back, creating a straight line from your head to your heels.

- Execute a push-up movement, bending your elbows and bringing your chest towards the wall.

- Return to the starting position and maintain a plank for 2-3 seconds. Repeat this sequence 8-10 times for a comprehensive workout.

Body Awareness Tips: Maintain a smooth connection with the wall throughout. Focus on stability and avoid any unnecessary movements.

Breath Tips: Sync your breathing naturally with the exercise. Inhale during the initiatory phase and exhale during exertion.

Safety Tips: Prioritize controlled movements over excessive force. Pay attention to your body's signals and avoid pushing beyond your comfort level.

Engaged Body Parts: Feel the engagement in your core, back, and arms. Ensure your shoulder blades are involved, and your legs play a role in maintaining balance.

2. Standing Wall Slide-Down

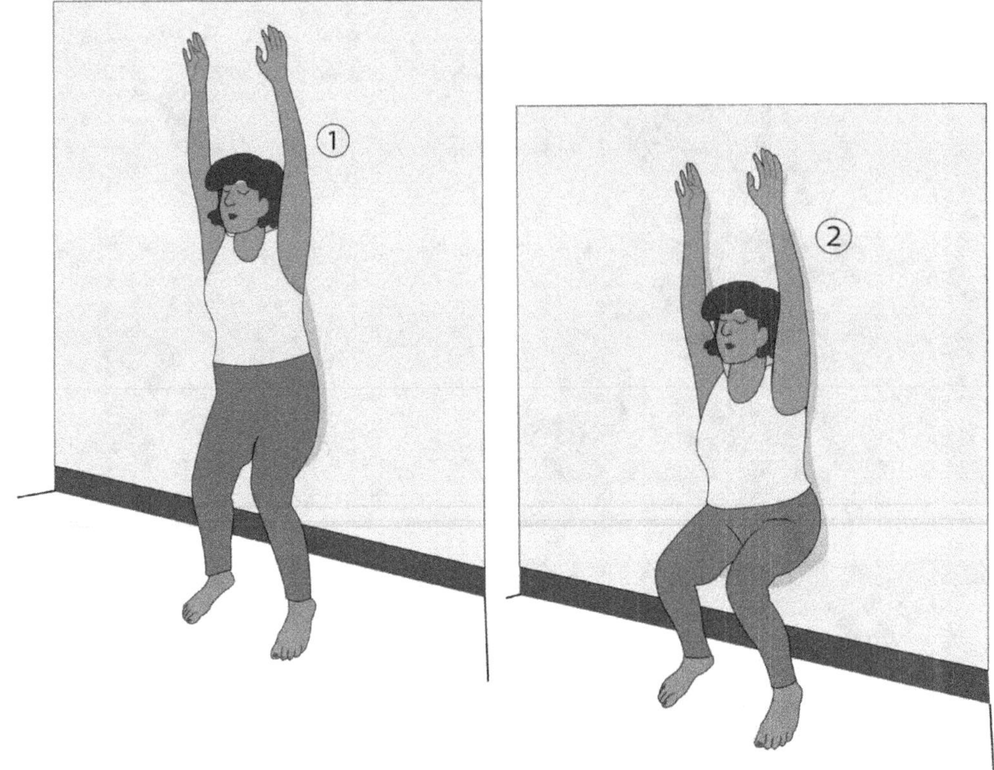

- Stand with your back against the wall, with your feet hip-width apart.
- Inhale, lifting your arms overhead.
- Exhale, slowly rolling down the wall, vertebra by vertebra, engaging your core.
- Inhale at the bottom, then exhale, rolling back up. Repeat 5-8 times.

Body Awareness Tips: Stay mindful of your body alignment against the wall. Focus on a gradual, controlled descent and ascent.

Breath Tips: Coordinate your breath with the movement. Inhale as you prepare and exhale during the descent and ascent.

Safety Tips: Avoid abrupt movements. Listen to your body, and if you feel discomfort, modify the range of motion accordingly.

Engaged Body Parts: Feel the engagement in your abdominal muscles and lower back, and ensure your arms are active throughout the exercise.

3. Wall Squat With Cushion Squeeze

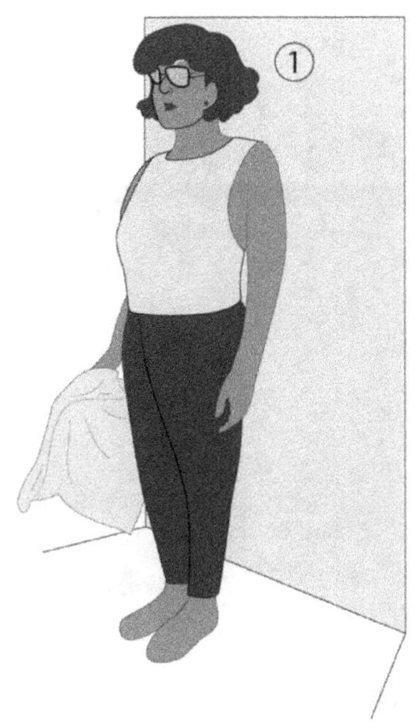 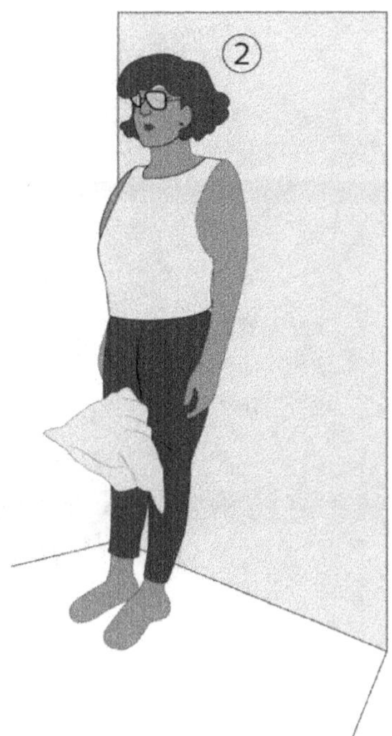 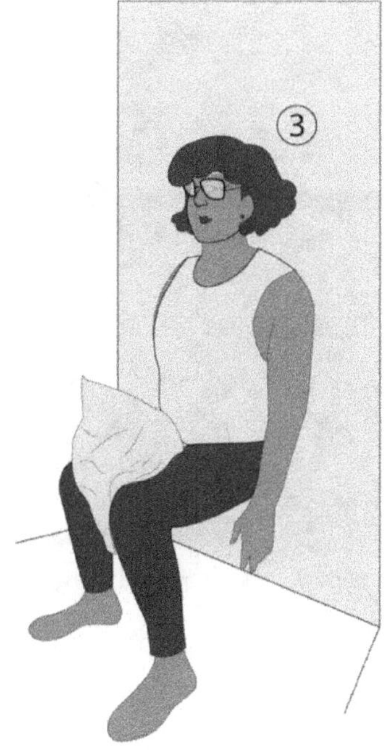

- Place a cushion between your knees, while standing with your back against the wall.

- Then, slide down the wall into a squat position, your knees bent at 90 degrees.

- Engage your core and squeeze the cushion with your knees, holding for 3-5 seconds.

- Release the squeeze and repeat 8-10 times.

Body Awareness Tips: Focus on maintaining a neutral spine against the wall. Be aware of your posture throughout the squat.

Breath Tips: Inhale as you lower into the squat, exhale as you engage your core and squeeze the cushion.

Safety Tips: Pay attention to your knee alignment; ensure they track over your toes during the squat. If you experience discomfort, adjust your range of motion.

Engaged Body Parts: Feel activation in your abdominal muscles, especially when squeezing the cushion. Also, sense engagement in your thighs and buttocks during the squat.

4. Forearm Push-Up

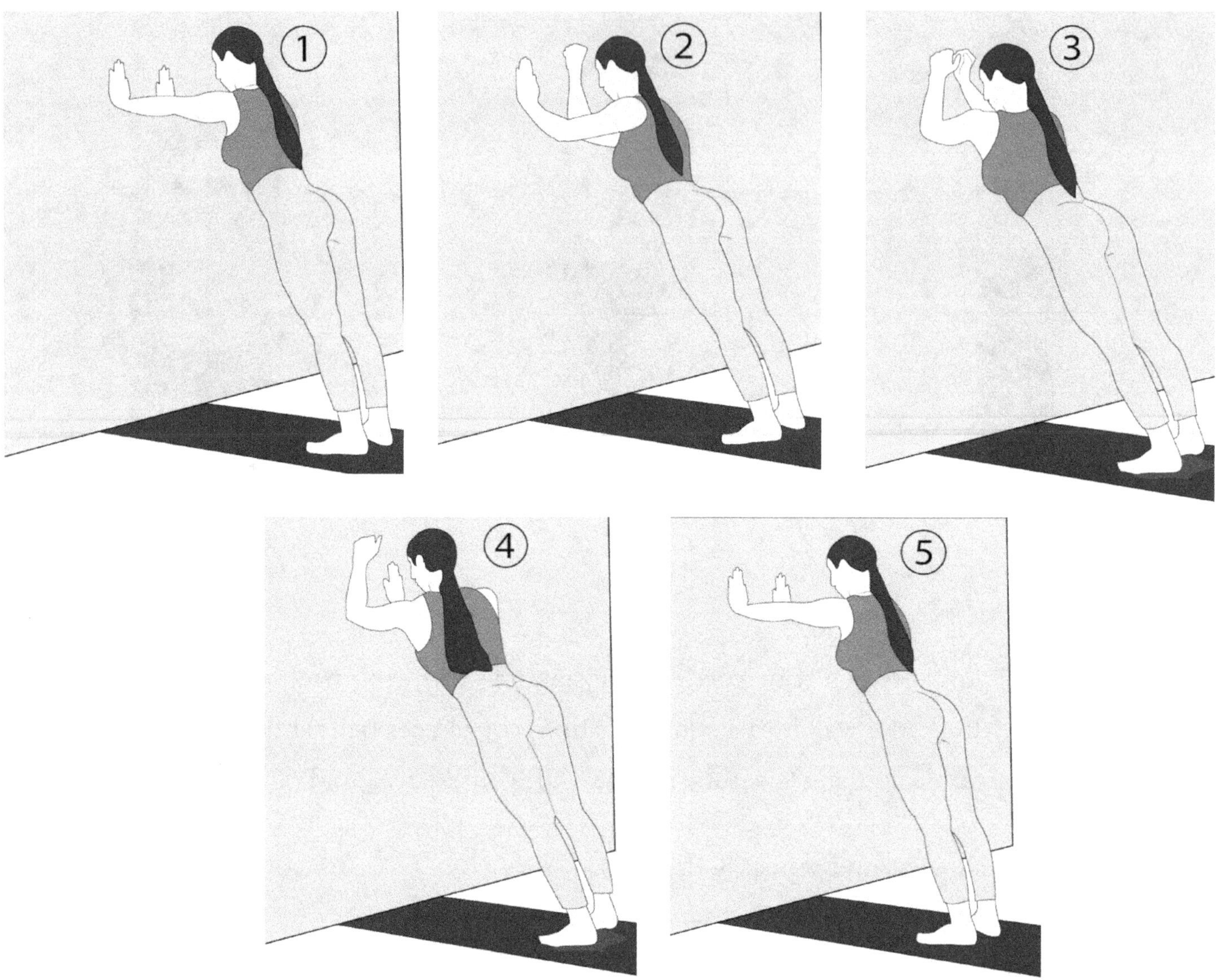

- You are standing a comfortable 20-30 inches from the wall, placing your hands on it, and extending your arms. Slightly lean forward, creating a gentle diagonal angle with your torso.

- Now, gently rest your right forearm on the wall while keeping your left arm extended. Feel the support. Then, with a seamless motion, lower your left forearm to join the right, transitioning into a plank against the wall on your forearms. Feel the strength in this position.

- Smoothly extend your right arm, effortlessly returning to the initial stance.

- Follow it up by extending your left arm, completing the cycle. Let's do this for a total of 10 times.

Body Awareness Tips: Pay special attention to how your torso aligns, ensuring it forms a straight line from your head to the heels throughout the movement.

Breath Tips: Inhale deeply as you gracefully lower into the forearm plank, and exhale with a sense of ease as you return. Keep your breath steady, like a comforting rhythm.

Safety Tips: Maintain a just-right distance from the wall, ensuring you find that sweet spot while avoiding any unnecessary strain on your wrists and shoulders.

Engaged Body Parts: Sense the power in your core, providing a steady anchor throughout the movement. Feel the engagement in your arms and shoulders, embracing the graceful flow of the exercise.

5. Wall Slide and Squat

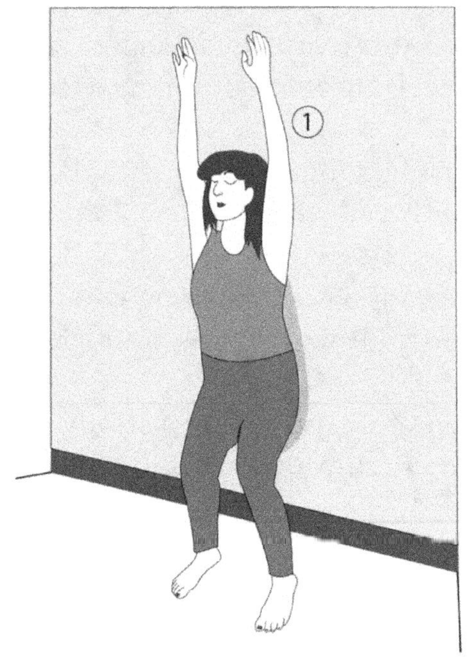
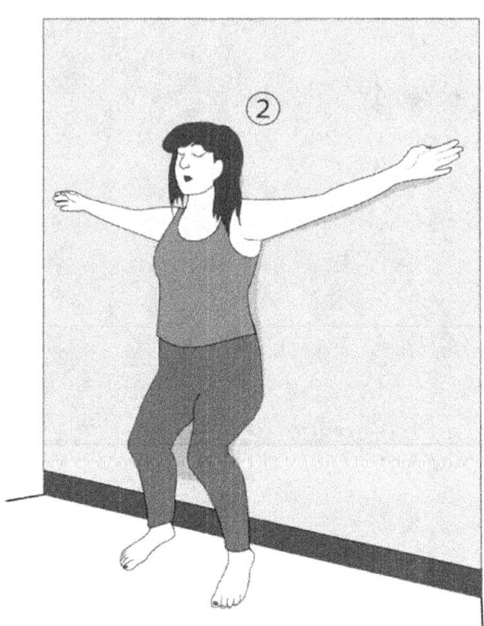

- Stand against the wall, feet hip-width apart.

- Inhale, raising arms overhead, fingertips touching the wall. (1)

- Exhale, bend your knees into a squat, slide your arms down until parallel to the floor. (2)

- Hold briefly, feeling the stretch, then inhale, straightening your knees and returning to the starting position.

- Repeat 8-10 times.

***

Body Awareness Tips: Pay attention to the alignment of your spine against the wall. Keep your core engaged throughout the movement.

Breath Tips: Inhale as you reach up, and exhale as you descend into the squat. Maintain a steady and controlled breath.

Safety Tips: Ensure your movements are controlled to prevent strain. If you feel any discomfort, modify the depth of your squat.

Engaged Body Parts: abdominals, deltoids (shoulder muscles), quadriceps, and hamstrings.

6. Wall Curl with Leg Extension

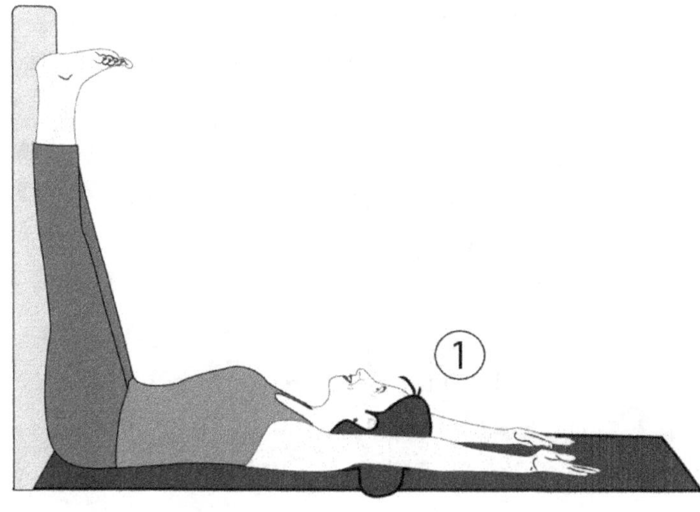

- Start by lying on your back with your legs fully extended against the wall and your arms stretched overhead. (1)

- Keep your abdomen contracted throughout the exercise.

- Without moving your legs, initiate a curl by bringing your arms forward towards the wall. (2)

- Engage your core as you perform the curl, feeling the contraction in your abdominal muscles.

- Return to the starting position with your arms extended overhead.

- Repeat this movement for 8-10 repetitions, focusing on controlled and deliberate curls.

Body Awareness Tips: Pay attention to how your body moves. Check your posture and feel the muscles at work.

Breath Tips: Inhale as you get ready, exhale during the curl, and then inhale again when extending. Sync your breath with your moves.

Safety Tips: Comfort is key. Make sure your setup feels right, and take it steady.

Engaged Body Parts: Core and legs. Get those muscles working together for a solid exercise.

7. Wall Reverse Twist Crunch

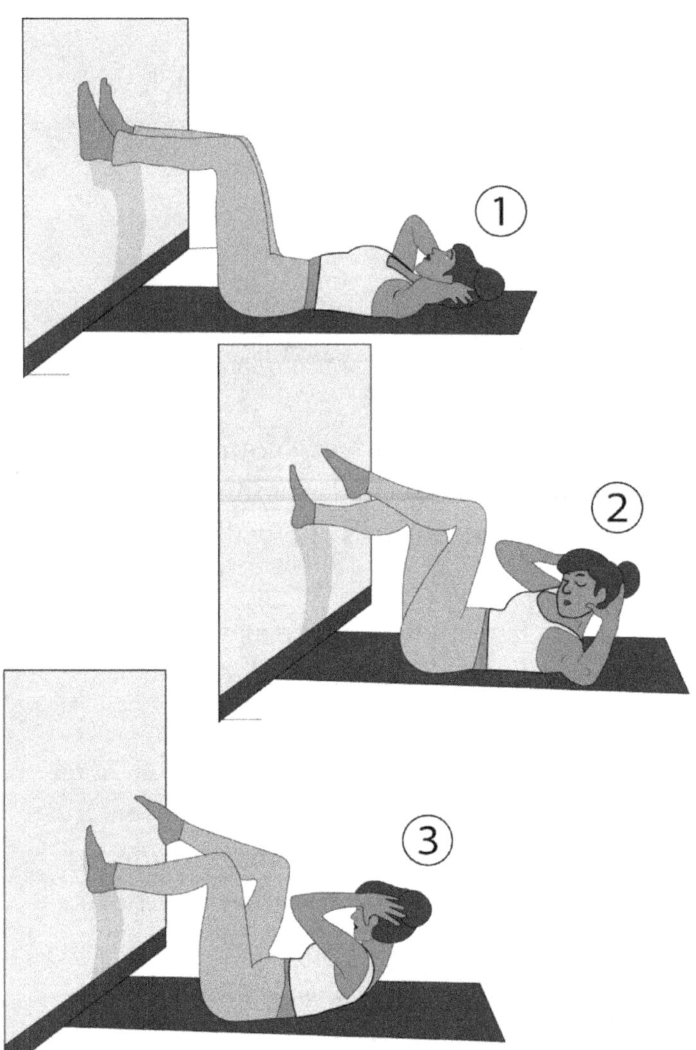

- Begin by lying down with your back on the mat, hands placed behind your neck, and elbows bent, resting on the ground. (1)

- Position your feet against the wall, with your legs forming a 90-degree angle.

- Engage your core muscles, then lift your head, neck, and shoulders off the mat, initiating a curl. (2)

- Twist your torso inch by inch to bring your right elbow toward your left knee. Return to the center and switch sides. (3)

- Keep alternating sides in a controlled and rhythmic motion. Aim for 10-15 repetitions on each side, increasing as you build strength.

Body Awareness Tips: Pay attention to the movement of your torso and feel the contraction in your obliques.

Breath Tips: Inhale as you prepare for the movement, exhale during the twist and curl, and inhale again as you return to the center.

Safety Tips: Ensure your neck is relaxed, and avoid pulling on it. Keep the movements controlled to protect your lower back.

Engaged Body Parts: Activate your abdominal muscles, especially the obliques, to execute the twist and curl effectively.

Chapter 6: Intermediate Wall Pilates Exercises

Welcome to a comprehensive exploration of different Wall Pilates targeted exercises, including the abdomen, back, legs, and buttocks. In the upcoming sections, in fact, we'll focus on specific exercises and insights crafted to boost strength, flexibility, and overall well-being in these targeted areas.

Let's delve into each section and discover ways to feel more connected and empowered throughout your body!

Abdomen Wall Pilates Exercises

1. Bridge Pose with Bent Knees

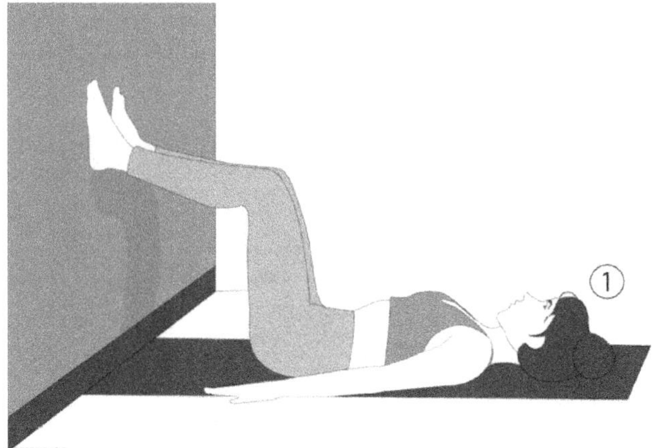

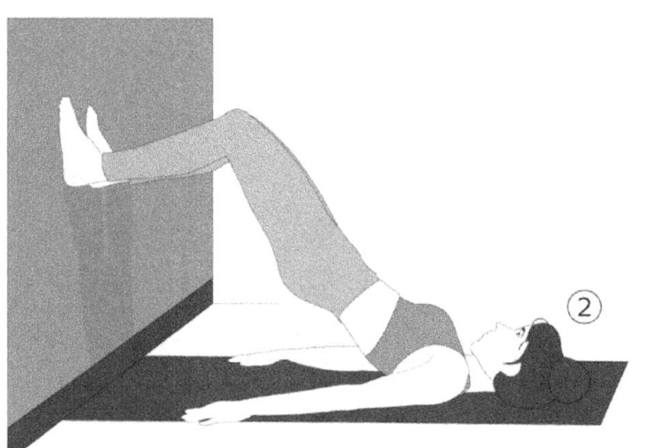

- First, lie down, stick your feet on the wall, and bend those knees at a comfy 90-degree angle. (1)

- Keep your hands close to your body, palms pressing into the floor. Pay attention to your spine, keep it neutral, and breathe naturally.

- Inhale when you're gearing up, and exhale as you lift your hips. Do not overextend; let's keep it smooth. (2)

- Engage those core muscles, glutes, and thighs for that perfect bridge position.

- Slowly lower those hips back to the floor, and don't forget to sync your breath with every move.

Body Awareness Tips: Watch that spine alignment and your feet against the wall. It's all about a steady foundation.

Breath Tips: Inhale the good vibes, exhale the stress. Keep it cool, steady, and controlled.

Safety Tips: Take it easy on your lower back; there is no need to rush. If it feels off, ease out of it, no pressure.

Engaged Body Parts: Activate those glutes, hamstrings, and core. Ground those shoulders, and let those arms play their supportive role.

2. Half-Arms Wheel

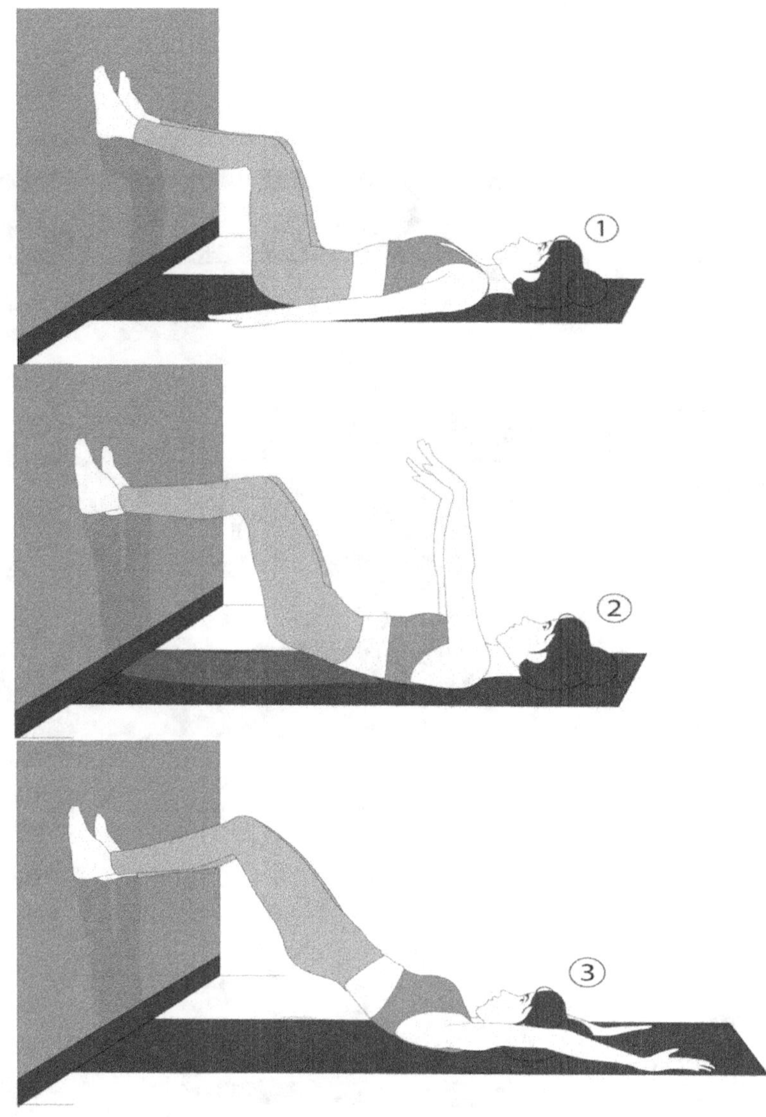

- Start in the same position as previous stretch, the bent-knee bridge, feet on the wall, hands close to the torso. (1)

- Now, elevate those arms like you're reaching for the stars and beyond (2)

- Lifting your butt a bit off the ground. (3)

- Slowly lower the arms and butt back to the start.

- Repeat this move five times for the full experience.

Body Awareness Tips: Keep that spine in check, and stay mindful the whole time.

Breath Tips: Inhale for the prep, exhale during the lift-off. Keep that breath rhythm going.

Safety Tips: Don't stretch too far, and let's keep those movements smooth. No need for lower back pain.

Engaged Body Parts: Core, glutes, and arms. Let the muscles do their thing for that stability and strength.

3. Point Your Toes

- Lie down, feet on the wall, legs are straight, toes flexed. Hands rest on the belly. (1)

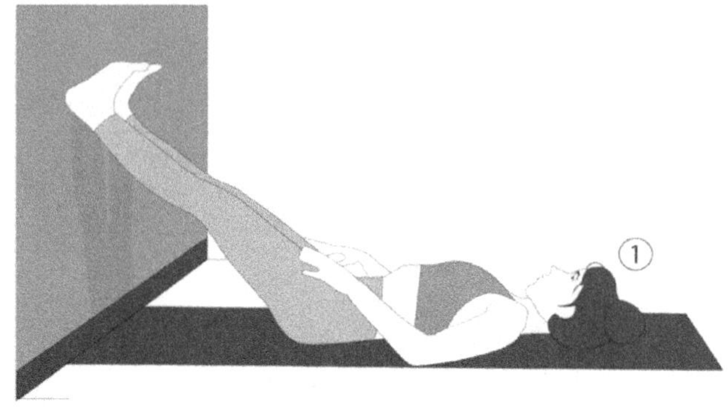

- Point those right toes and point your hands down on the floor while lifting the booty a bit. Keep the left foot on the wall. (2)

- While pointing your toes, feel the stretch in your right leg, especially in the back of the thigh. Keep your left foot against the wall for that extra support.

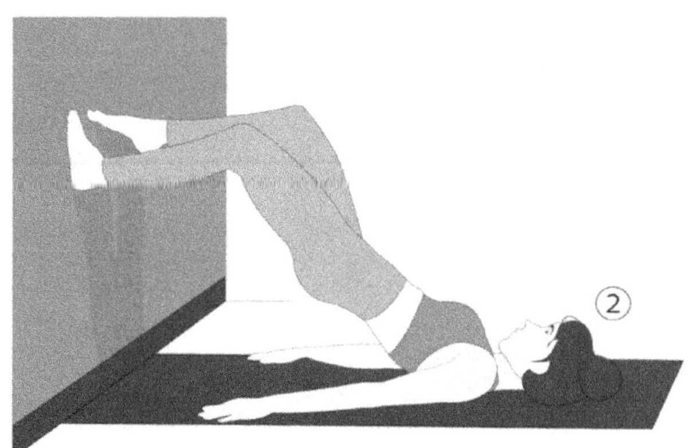

- Return to the starting position, allowing your buttocks to settle, inch by inch. Keep this toe-pointing movement going for five rounds on each leg.

- If you want to take it further, you can also keep your body as it is during the moment when you point your toes, bending your right leg to create a 90-degree angle but bringing your knee closer to your face. Hold for 5 seconds, then return to the starting position and repeat on the other side. (3)

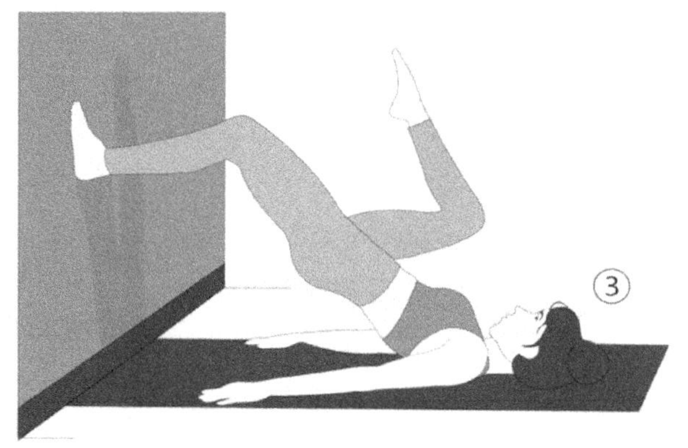

Body Awareness Tips: Torso stability is the key. Feel those lower-body vibes.

Breath Tips: Inhale the good vibes, exhale as you lift. Keep it steady, in and out.

Safety Tips: Easy on the neck and shoulders. If it feels weird, tweak the move or check with a fitness bud.

Engaged Body Parts: Activate the core, lower abs, and those butt muscles. Feel the leg vibes with each toe point.

4. Arms Movements

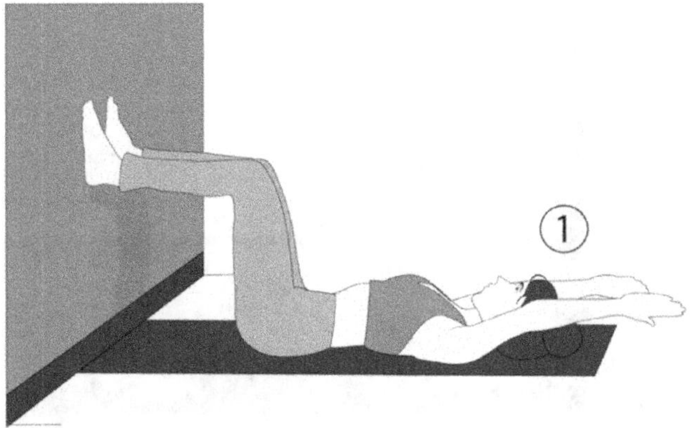

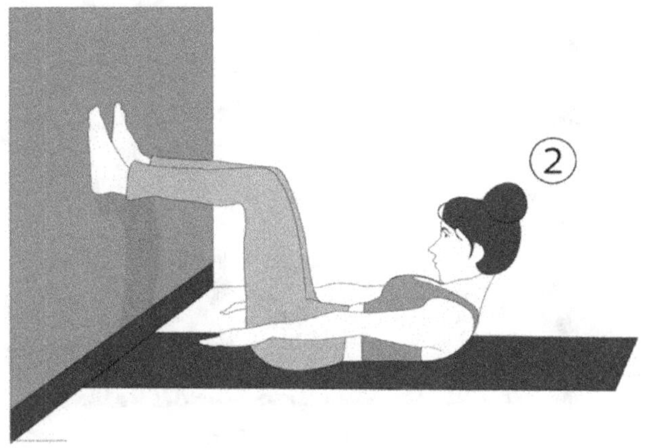

- Lie down, feet on the wall, and bend those knees.

- Inhale, raise your hands above your head. (1)

- Exhale, bring them back down, lifting the torso but keeping that spine in a chill zone. Ten rounds, let's go. (2)

Body Awareness Tips: Shoulders lead the way, and that spine is your buddy. Keep it steady.

Breath Tips: Inhale and reach for the skies. Exhale, back down. Find your personal breath rhythm and go with it.

Safety Tips: No strain on the neck, please. If things feel off, adjust the move or get a second opinion.

Engaged Body Parts: Shoulders are in the spotlight. Core's got your back. Keep it all controlled and intentional.

5. Forearm Plank with Feet on the Wall

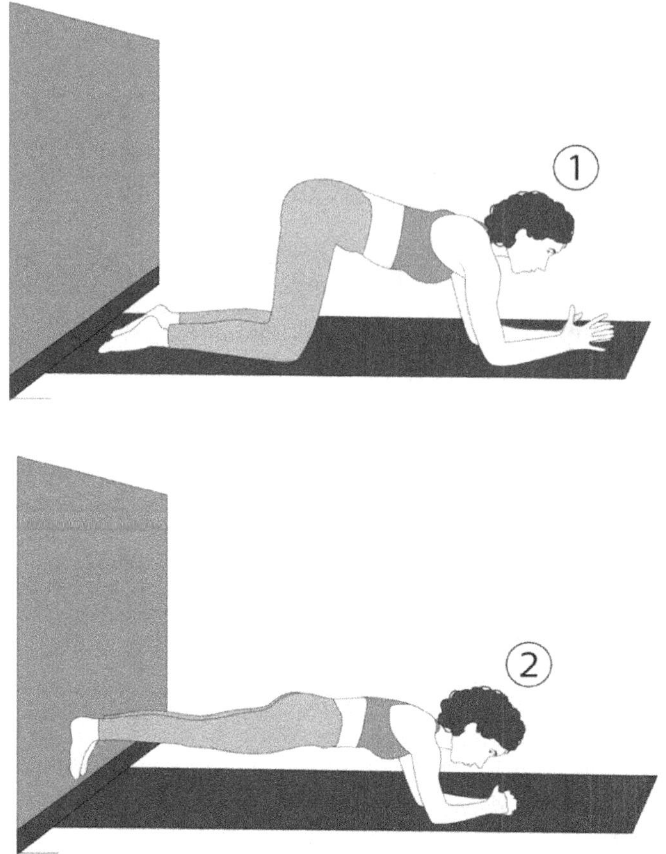

- Get on all fours - hands and knees touching the ground and neutral spine, forearms on the floor. (1)
- Head level with the ground and feet on the wall. (2)
- Hold that plank pose for 30 to 45 seconds, from head to heel.

Body Awareness Tips: Keep that core strong and your spine in check. It's all about that straight line.

Breath Tips: Inhale the good vibes, exhale the stress. Steady breaths, in through the nose, out through the mouth.

Safety Tips: No dipping hips or arching backs. Keep those wrists and elbows in sync. If it gets heavy, ease up a bit.

Engaged Body Parts: The core is your center, steering the ship. Shoulders, arms, and the spine are all in on this.

Legs and Buttocks Wall Pilates Exercises

6. Legs in the sky

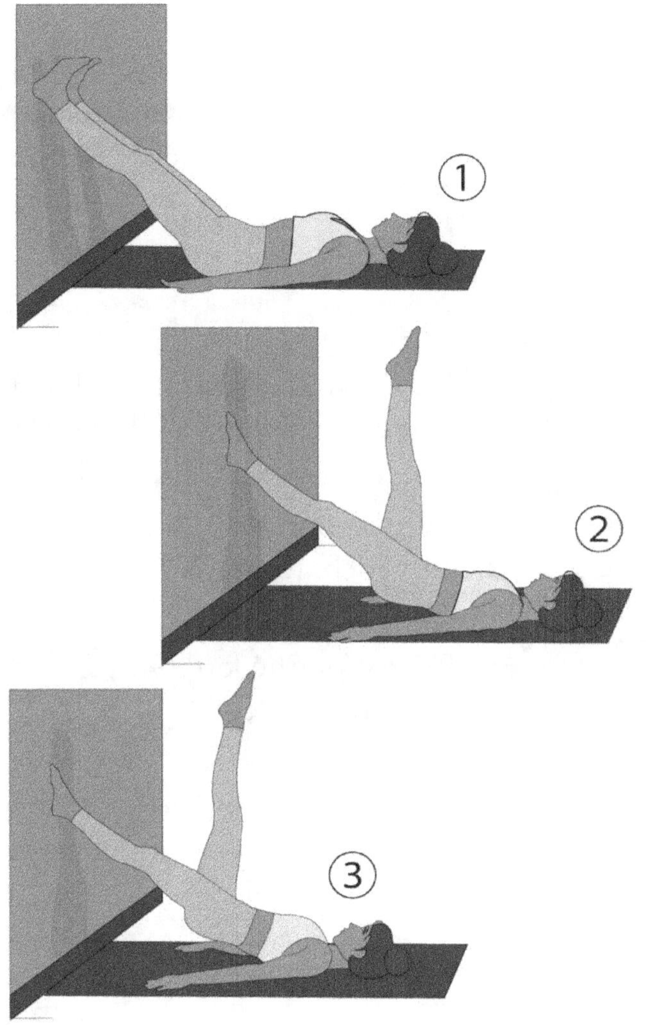

- Lie down, feet on the wall, legs are straight, toes flexed, and hands on the floor. (1)

- Lift the right leg and butt, inch by inch. Slowly lower. (2) – (3)

- Repeat on the left side. Alternate for five times on each leg.

Body Awareness Tips: Feel each leg's journey. Keep that core engaged, and let your back feel the floor.

Breath Tips: Inhale on the lift, exhale on the lower. Nice and steady, no need to rush.

Safety Tips: No sudden moves, and let that back be cozy on the ground. If things feel off, take it easy.

Engaged Body Parts: The core, lower abs, and those butt muscles are in the spotlight. Enjoy the lift and descent.

7. Leg in the Sky 90 Degrees

It's a similar drill to the previous exercise, but let's aim for that sweet 90-degree angle.

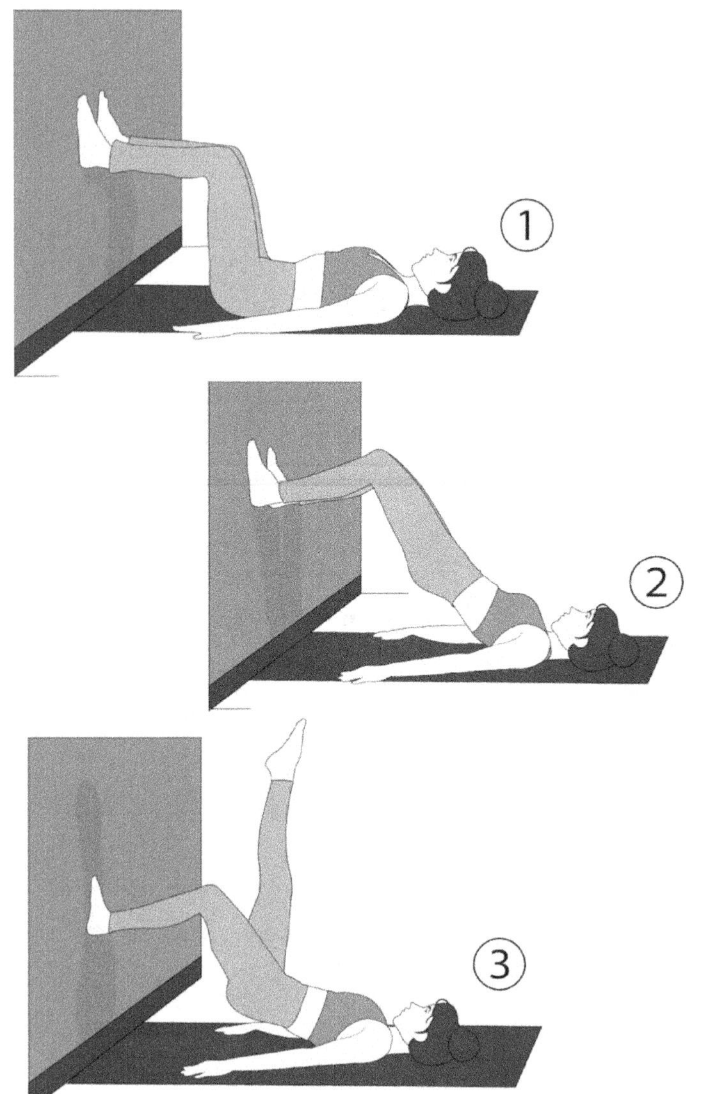

- Lie down, feet on the wall, but this time, your knees are bent. (1)

- Lift the butt, then the right leg, inch by inch. (2) – (3)

- Repeat on the left. Go for five rounds on each leg.

Body Awareness Tips: Focus on that gradual lift. Check-in with your feet against the wall.

Breath Tips: Inhale for the lift, exhale for the descent. Match that breath with your moves.

Safety Tips: Back comfort is key. No abrupt moves.

Engaged Body Parts: Glutes, thighs, and core. Keep that core stability going

8. Leg Circles

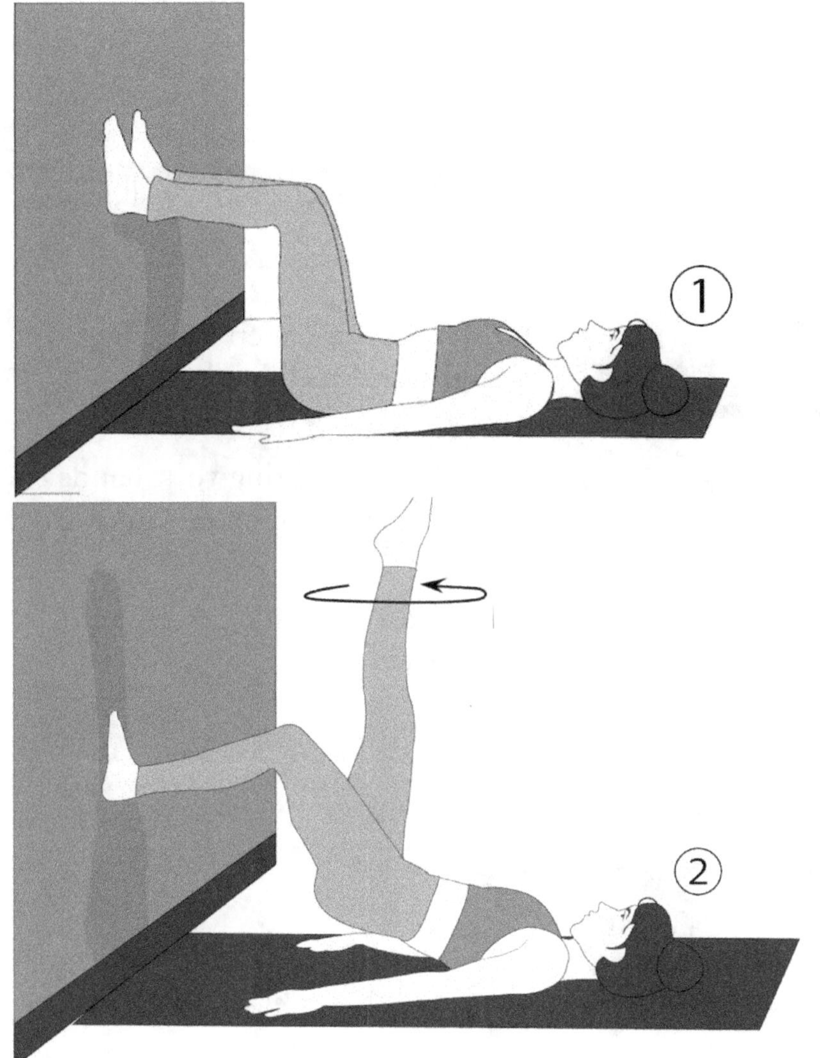

- Lie down, feet on the wall, knees bent. (1)

- Lift the butt, raise that right leg, and add some leg circles. (2)

- Slowly lower, inch by inch, keeping the core engaged.

- Repeat on the left.

- Five circles on each leg, and we're grooving!

Body Awareness Tips: Feel that lower back and hips groove in the circles. Keep it smooth.

Breath Tips: Inhale, lift, and start the circle. Exhale, finish the circle. Keep it in sync.

Safety Tips: No rush and keep that back comfy. If it's not feeling right, dial it down a bit.

Engaged Body Parts: Glutes, thighs: keep it all controlled.

9. Bridge Pose with Straight Legs

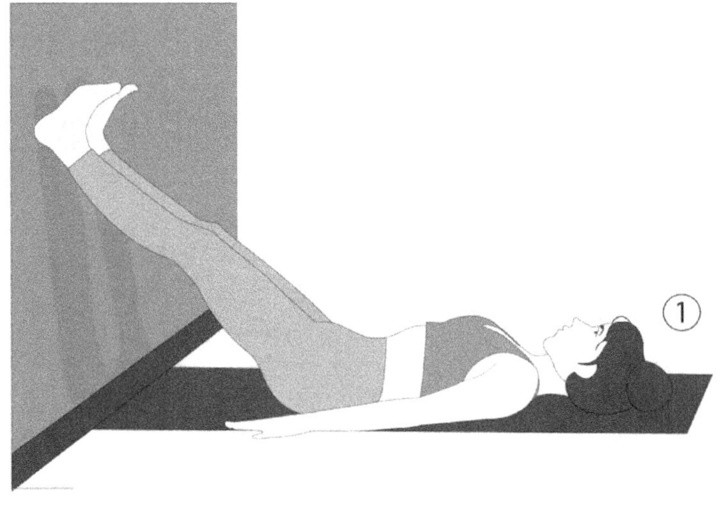

- Lie down, feet on the wall, legs straight. (1)

- Lift that butt, keep those legs straight, and feel that bridge. (2)

- You can also bring your hands on your glutes for extra support.

- Hold for 4 breaths, then lower back down.

- Repeat 2 times.

Body Awareness Tips: Straight and stable, that's the goal. Keep tabs on that lower body.

Breath Tips: Inhale for the prep, exhale for the lift. Keep that breath steady.

Safety Tips: Easy on the neck and shoulders. If it feels off, adjust the move or check with a fitness professional.

Engaged Body Parts: The core, lower abs, and glutes are the heroes here. Embrace the lift.

10. Wall-Plow Pose

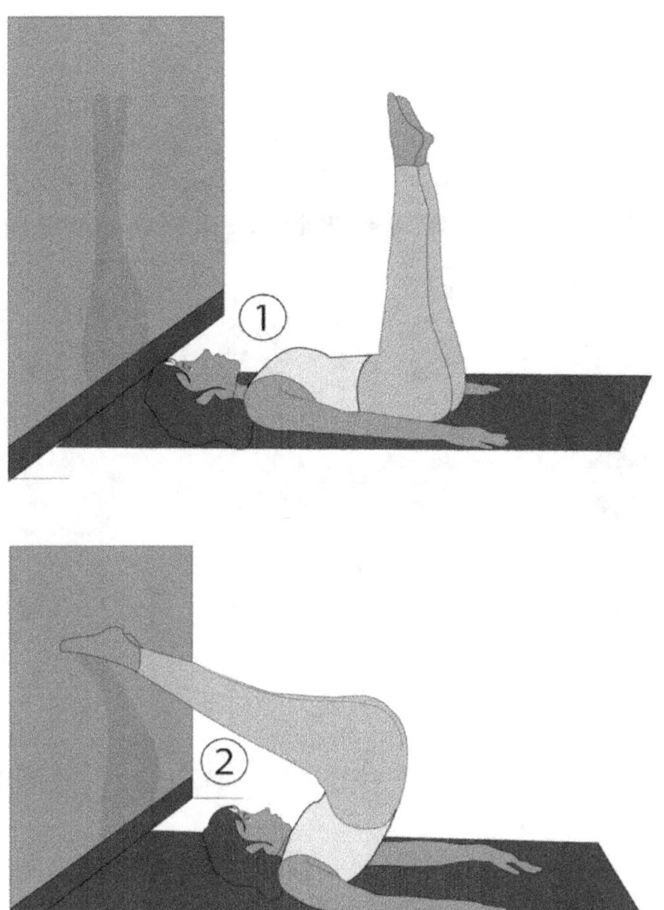

- Lie down, head close to the wall, legs up at a 90-degree angle. (1)
- Lift those legs and touch the wall with your toes. (2)
- Repeat five times, like a graceful wall dancer.

Body Awareness Tips: Smooth and controlled—feel the alignment of your spine and neck.

Breath Tips: Inhale the lift, exhale the touch. Keep that breath in harmony with your moves.

Safety Tips: Comfort is key; there is no need to force the wall to touch.

Engaged Body Parts: Core is your buddy here. Feel those abs engage as you lift and touch that wall.

Back Wall Pilates Exercises

11. Tilt Forward

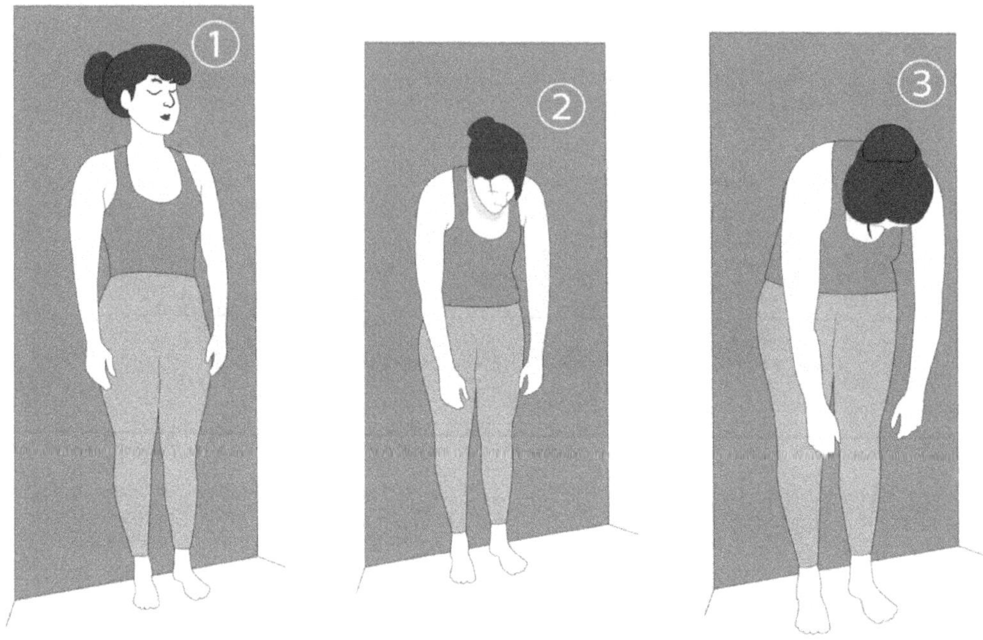

- Keep your back straight against the wall, heels and butt touching, hands crossed over, and palms facing in. (1)

- Now, the slow tilt forward begins. Round that spine, let the arms follow suit, but keep those heels and that butt glued to the wall. (2) – (3)

- Hold the tilt for a zen-like count of 10 breaths, and then gently ease back to the start.

Body Awareness Tips: Feel the entire length of your spine as you tilt. Keep an eye on those heels and the connection with the wall for a stable posture.

Breath Tips: Inhale the calm, exhale the tension. Find a rhythm that complements your tilt, making each breath intentional and relaxed.

Safety Tips: No need to push too hard; let the tilt be gentle. Ensure your back is comfortable, and if it's not, adjust the range of the tilt accordingly.

Engaged Body Parts: Your core is in play here—feel those abdominal muscles working to maintain the connection. The spine and arms also get in on the action, creating a harmonious tilt.

12. Foundation Training Bridge

This is a variation of the bridge pose, coming from Foundation Training.

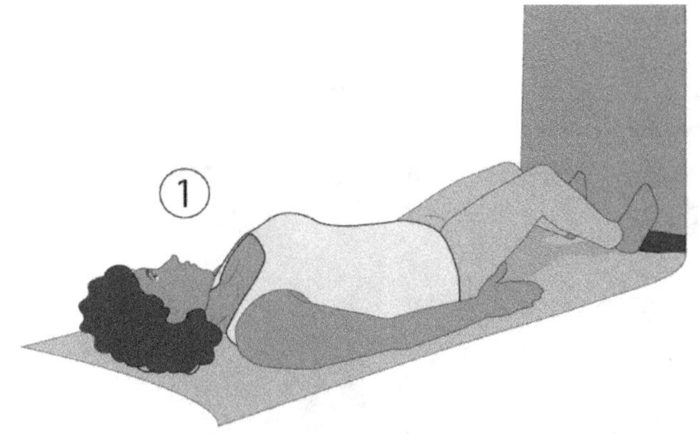

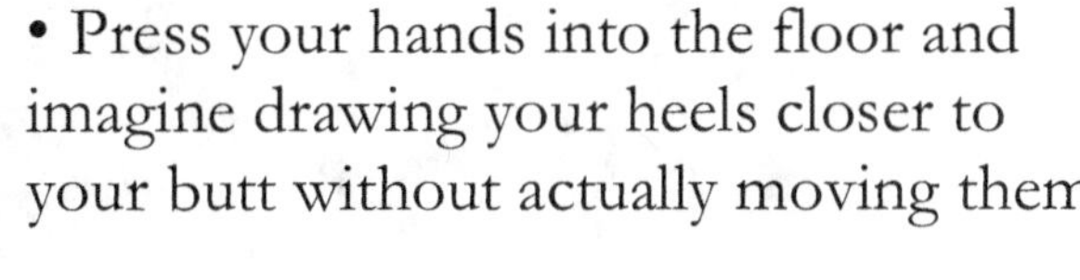

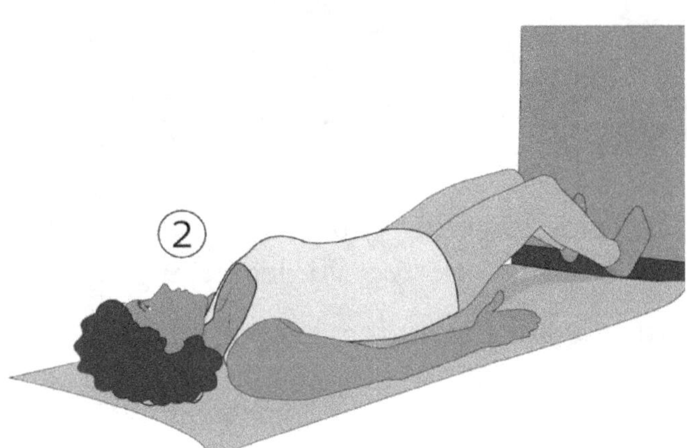

• Start with your heels touching the wall, lying on your back with hands across your body and palms facing inwards. (1)

• Gently lift your butt a few inches off the floor, ensuring your heels stay connected to the wall. (2)

• Press your hands into the floor and imagine drawing your heels closer to your butt without actually moving them.

• Hold this position for 15 seconds, feeling the engagement in your glutes and lower back, then slowly release back down. Repeat this sequence for a total of 5 times.

Body Awareness Tips: Tune into the subtle movements in your lower back and hips as you lift and press. Focus on the connection between your heels and the wall for stability.

Breath Tips: Inhale as you prepare to lift, exhale as you press your hands into the floor, and maintain a steady breath throughout the hold. Use your breath to enhance the mind-body connection.

Safety Tips: Be mindful of the intensity in your lower back; if you feel any strain, reduce the range of motion. Ensure your neck and shoulders remain relaxed on the ground.

Engaged Body Parts: Feel the activation in your glutes and lower your back muscles as you lift and press. Your core will also play a role in stabilizing this variation of the Bridge pose.

13. Wall-sitting with Raised Knees

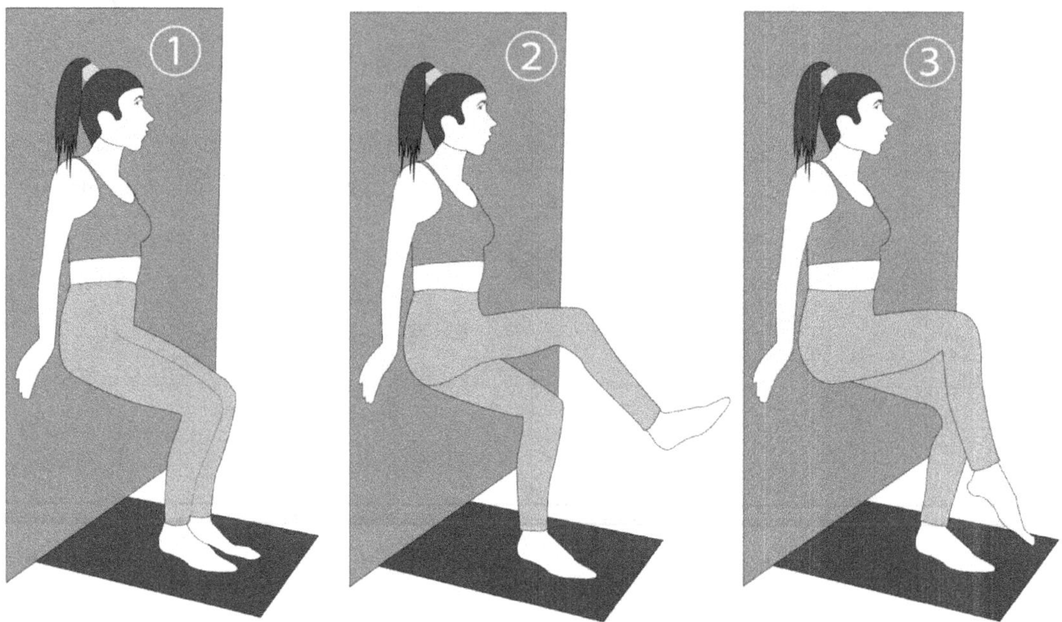

- Get cozy with your back against the wall. Imagine lowering yourself into that comfy chair, hips parallel to the ground, and knees forming a perfect 90-degree angle. (1)

- Engage that core of yours and gracefully lift one knee at a time, keeping them gently bent. (2)

- Return to your starting position and switch legs.

- Keep the flow going, alternating for a total of 10 reps on each leg.

Body Awareness Tips: Tune into how your hips and knees align—keep them parallel to the ground. Feel the subtle engagement in your core, and make friends with the stability of your posture against the wall.

Breath Tips: Inhale the good vibes as you sink into your imaginary chair, and exhale as each leg takes its turn to shine. Let your breath dance in harmony with your movements, creating a mindful rhythm.

Safety Tips: Take it easy on your knees, ensuring the movement is smooth and under control. If anything feels off, especially in those knees or lower back, take it down a notch and adjust the range of motion.

Engaged Body Parts: Your core steals the spotlight as each leg gets its moment. Quadriceps and glutes ensure a solid connection with the wall for added stability.

14. Side Bend

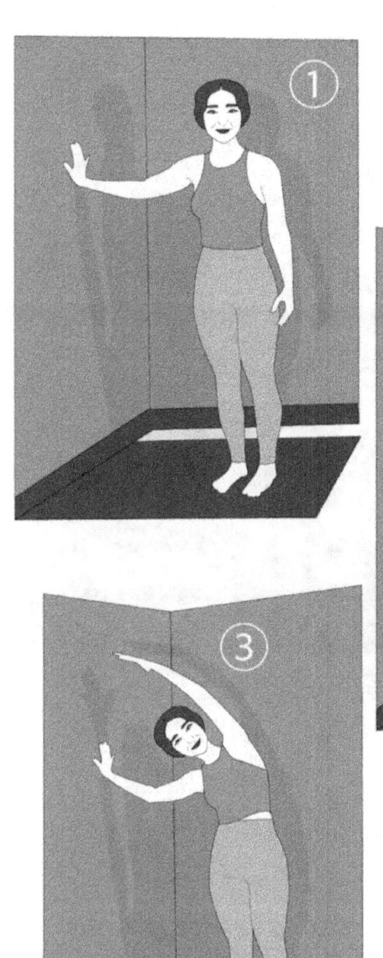

- Place your right hand against the wall, keeping your arm slightly bent. (1)

- Indulge in a graceful side bend to the right side, extending your left hand to touch the wall. (2)

- Ensure your torso stands firm—no rounding or unnecessary movements. Keep that left shoulder gracefully over the right one. (3)

- Repeat this delightful stretch to the other side. 5 repetitions on each side.

Body Awareness Tips: Pay attention to your torso's alignment. Feel the stretch in your side body without compromising the stability of your shoulders, maintaining a straight and supported posture.

Breath Tips: Inhale deeply as you prepare for the bend, and exhale smoothly as you lean to the side.

Safety Tips: Be gentle on your torso—no abrupt twists or overextensions. If you sense any strain, ease off the stretch. The key here is a controlled and mindful side bend that feels good for your body.

Engaged Body Parts: Your obliques take center stage as they elongate and contract during the side bend. Feel the engagement in your arms and shoulders, maintaining stability with the support of the wall.

15. Seated Forward Fold

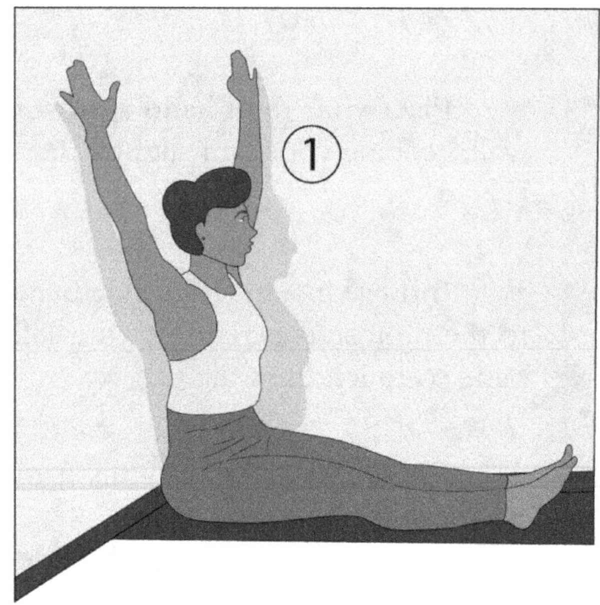
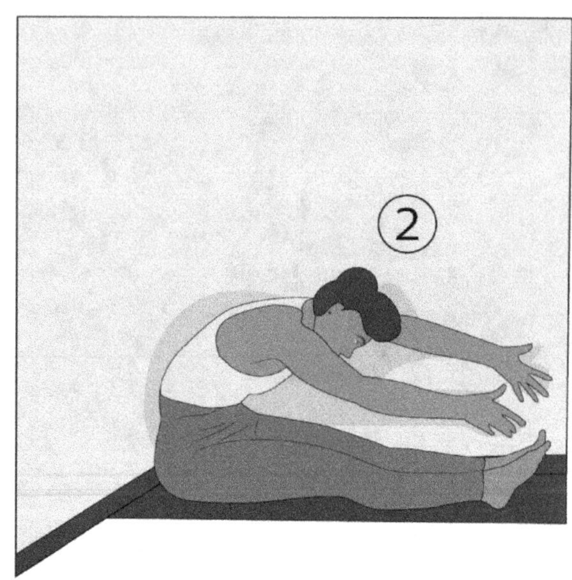

- Find a comfortable seated position with your back against the wall and hands up above the head. (1)

- As you embark on a soothing forward fold, reach towards your toes, allowing your back to move gently. (2)

- Immerse yourself in this stretch, staying in the pose for a tranquil 10 breaths.

Body Awareness Tips: Cultivate awareness of your spine and the gentle curve as you fold forward. Feel the lengthening in your hamstrings and lower back, ensuring a gradual and mindful descent.

Breath Tips: Inhale deeply, inviting a sense of space and openness. Exhale slowly, releasing tension and allowing your body to surrender into the stretch.

Safety Tips: Approach the forward fold with gentleness; avoid pushing your body beyond its comfort. If you feel any discomfort, ease back slightly.

Engaged Body Parts: Sense the stretch in your hamstrings and the gentle activation in your lower back. Let your arms and shoulders gracefully reach towards your toes, fostering a sense of length and release in your upper body. It's a serene unfolding of both body and breath.

Upper Body and Shoulder Wall Pilates Exercises

16. Cactus Arms

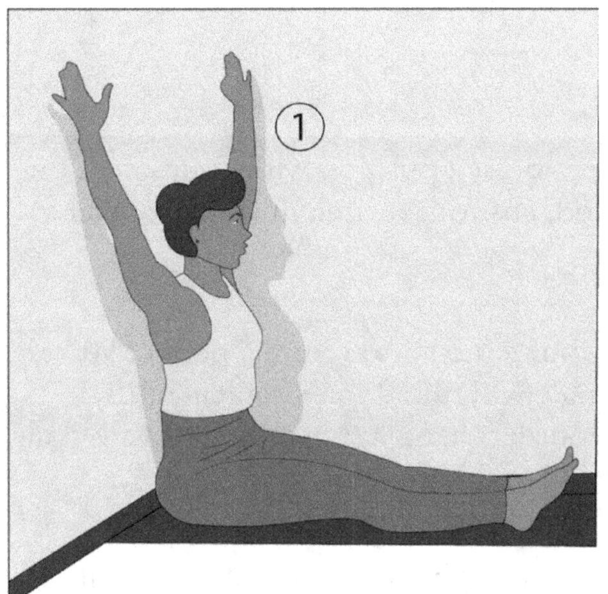 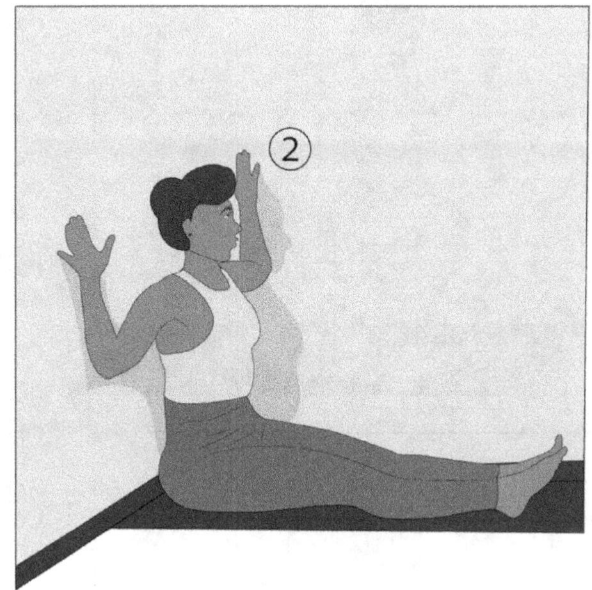

- In a relaxed seated position with your back against the wall, start with your hands raised above your head, taking a deep inhale. Engage the core. (1)

- As you exhale, maintain contact with the wall and gracefully lower your arms into a cactus shape. (2)

- Repeat this fluid motion for a rejuvenating set of 10 repetitions.

Body Awareness Tips: Heighten your awareness of the alignment of your spine against the wall. Feel the controlled descent of your arms, ensuring a smooth and deliberate movement.

Breath Tips: Inhale deeply before the movement, preparing for the graceful lowering of your arms. Exhale slowly and rhythmically as you create the cactus shape. Sync your breath with the serene flow of your arms.

Safety Tips: Prioritize a gentle and controlled descent of your arms, avoiding sudden movements. If you experience any discomfort, reduce the range of motion. Embrace the motion with ease, allowing it to be a comforting stretch.

Engaged Body Parts: Sense the engagement in your shoulders and upper back as you lower your arms. Feel the stretch across your chest in the cactus position, enhancing both flexibility and posture.

17. 180 Degrees

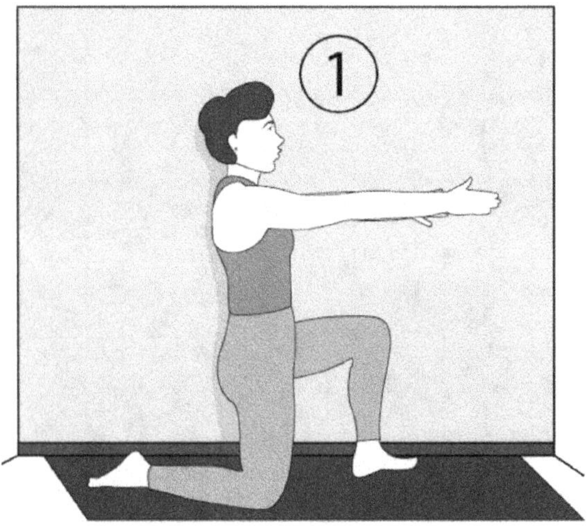

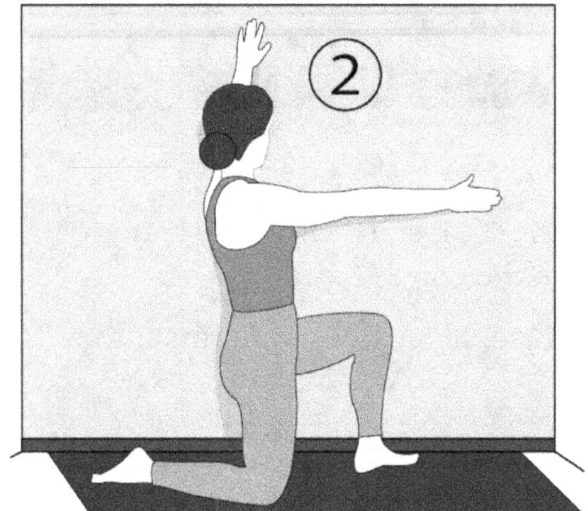

- Start in a poised position with your knees on the ground, ensuring a straight spine parallel to the wall.

- Point your left foot to create a perfect 90-degree angle with the floor, simultaneously placing your left hand against the wall with your arm parallel to the wall. (1)

- Elevate your right arm to shoulder height, parallel to the floor, with your hand facing inward.

- From this starting point, maintaining stability, glide your left hand against the wall while rounding the shoulder. (2)

- This action turns your torso to face the wall, guiding your arm to reach behind you. (3)

- Return to the initial position and gracefully repeat this movement for a revitalizing set of 7 repetitions.

- Subsequently, switch sides and perform the same sequence.

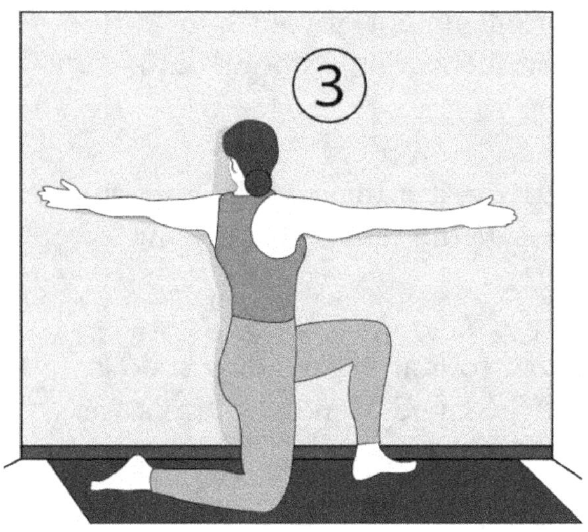

Body Awareness Tips: Heighten your awareness of body alignment; ensure your spine remains straight and parallel to the wall throughout the movement. Feel the controlled rotation of your torso.

Breath Tips: Inhale deeply as you prepare for the movement, and exhale slowly and steadily as you slide your hand along the wall. Sync your breath with the graceful rotation.

Safety Tips: Prioritize a smooth and controlled motion, avoiding any abrupt movements that may strain your shoulder. If you feel discomfort, modify the range of motion or consult with a professional.

Engaged Body Parts: Sense the engagement in your core and shoulders as you rotate, maintaining a stable foundation with your knees on the ground. Feel the stretch and flexibility in your upper body, promoting both strength and mobility.

18. 180 Reverse

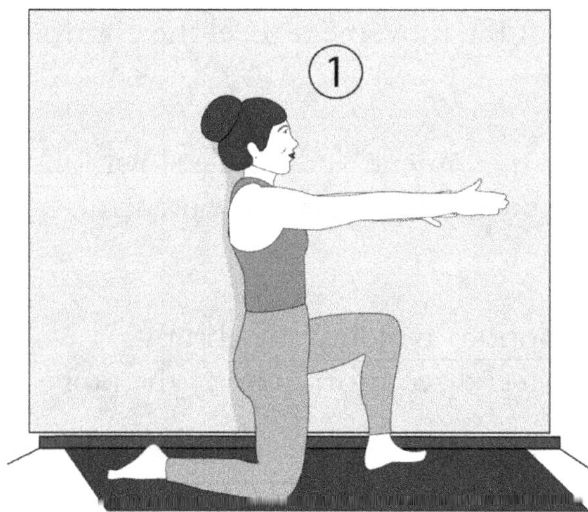

- Start by kneeling with a straight back, facing the wall.

- Point your left foot to the side, raising both arms to shoulder height with your palms facing in. (1)

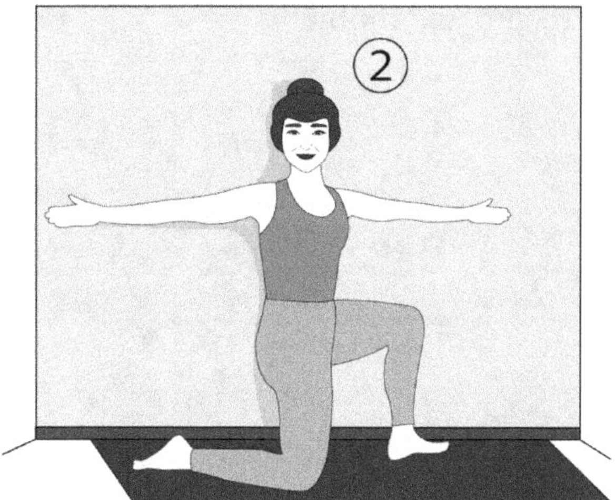

- Now, while keeping your left arm in place, smoothly rotate your right arm outward, turning your torso to the right. (2)

- Imagine drawing a long line with your arms. Return to the starting point and switch sides, repeating the process.

Body Awareness Tips: Pay attention to your posture, keeping your back straight as you move. Focus on the gentle rotation of your torso.

Breath Tips: Breathe naturally, but try to exhale as you twist, syncing your breath with the movement.

Safety Tips: Keep the motion controlled to avoid strain. If it feels uncomfortable, adjust the range of motion or seek guidance.

Engaged Body Parts: Feel your core and shoulders working as you gracefully turn your torso. Enjoy the stretch in your upper body, building strength and flexibility.

19. Push Up Internal Hands Rotation

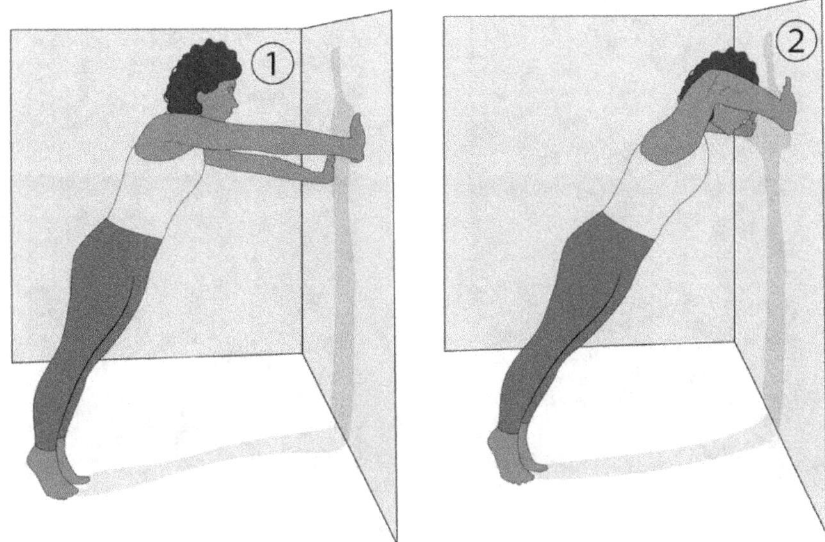

- Get into position by placing your hands on the wall, arms fully extended, and positioning your feet 20-30 inches away from the wall. (1)
- Now, it's push-up time, but here's the twist – literally. Rotate your hands internally as you push up. (2)
- Repeat this move for a full set.

Body Awareness Tips: Focus on maintaining a straight line from your head down to your heels, and make friends with your core muscles for that extra stability. Don't forget to notice the subtle rotation of your hands with each push-up.

Breath Tips: Inhale the good stuff as you lower your chest towards the wall, and exhale the effort as you push back up. Keep that breath flowing smoothly for optimal control.

Safety Tips: Comfort is key. Make sure there's a sweet spot between your hands and the wall. If your wrists or shoulders aren't feeling the love, tweak your hand placement. Listen to what your body's telling you, and avoid going into overdrive.

Engaged Body Parts: Feel the collaboration between your chest, shoulders, triceps, and your trusty core during each push-up. The internal hand rotation adds a bit of flair, getting different muscle groups in on the action for a workout that covers all the bases.

20. Hand on the Back of the Head

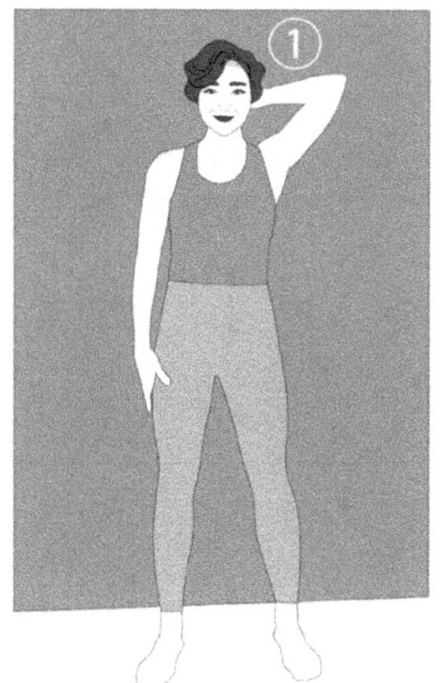
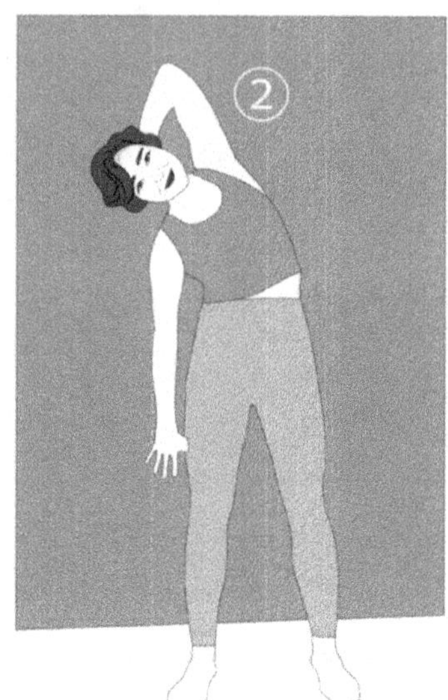

- Get cozy with the wall, ensuring your back is snug against it, and align your chin parallel to the floor.

- Now, take your left hand and place it behind your nape against the wall, with the elbow soaring higher than your head. (1)

- From this starting position, tilt your head over to the right, keeping that arm and hand rock-steady. (2)

- Straighten up, rinse, and repeat this delightful head tilt ten times before swapping sides.

Body Awareness Tips: Pay attention to the smooth movement of your head and arm, ensuring they dance together harmoniously against the wall.

Breath Tips: Inhale the goodness as you set up, exhale with grace as you tilt your head. Breathe in a relaxed rhythm to enhance the flow of each movement.

Safety Tips: Let comfort lead the way. If any part of this feels off-kilter or uncomfortable, adjust the position. Always prioritize the well-being of your neck and spine.

Engaged Body Parts: Your left arm is the star here, working in tandem with your neck. Feel the subtle engagement in your shoulder and arm as you gracefully tilt your head, creating a delightful stretch.

Total Body Wall Pilates Exercises

21. Tap the Toes

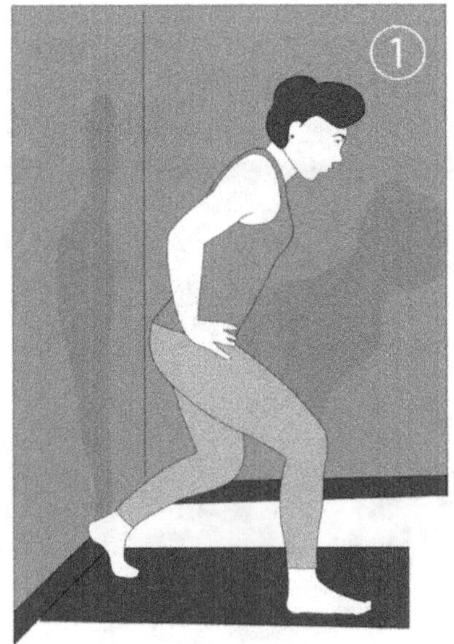 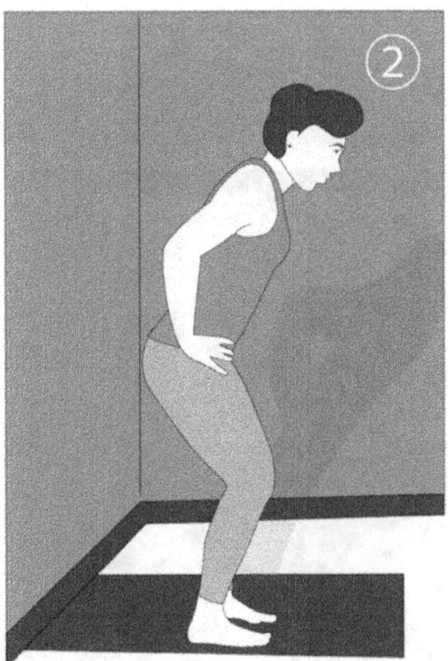

- Plant yourself by the wall, hands confidently on your hips, shoulder-width apart, and bend those knees a little. Take your left calf and let it cozy up against the wall while your right foot stands its ground. (1)

- Without stirring the rest of your body or that steadfast right leg, delicately reach your left foot towards the right one, tapping the toes on the ground. (2)

- Swap sides with finesse. Your right calf now gets its turn against the wall, and your left foot takes center stage.

- Keep this elegant dance going, alternating sides for a total of 10 times each.

Body Awareness Tips: Your body is the hero of this story. Pay heed to its alignment, ensuring that each graceful toe-tap is a symphony of movement.

Breath Tips: Inhale the promise of each toe-tap, exhale with the satisfaction of a gentle stretch. Let your breath be your companion, flowing seamlessly with each movement.

Safety Tips: Listen to your body's cues. If anything feels amiss or uncomfortable, adjust the distance from the wall or modify the movement. Your comfort is the key.

Engaged Body Parts: Feel the subtle engagement in your calves, the gentle stretch in your legs, and the stability in your hips.

22. Straight and Bent

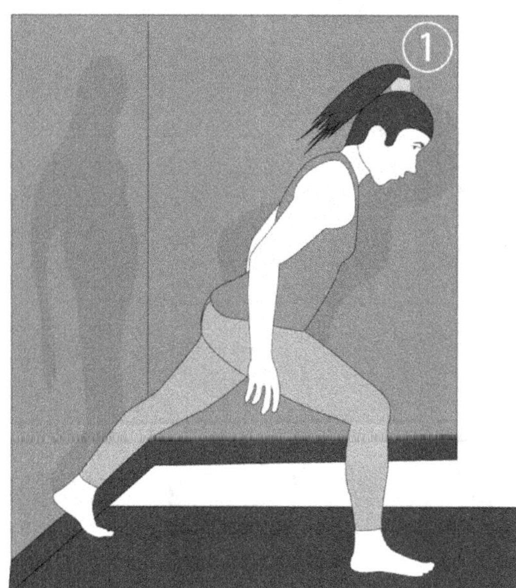 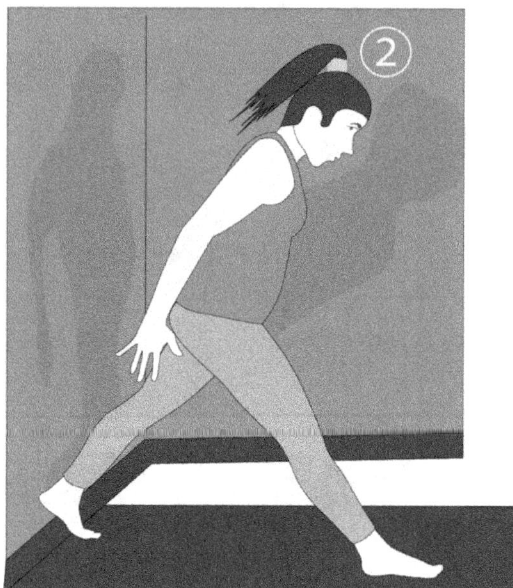

- Stand about 20 inches away from the wall, with your right knee bent and the left one straight, left calf gently touching the wall while your right foot stays firm on the ground. (1)

- Now, without moving your upper body, gracefully straighten and bend that right leg. (2)

- Repeat this interplay 10 times, then smoothly switch sides.

Body Awareness Tips: This is your body's own choreography. Tune in to how each straightening and bending movement feels, ensuring a mindful motion.

Breath Tips: Inhale the anticipation of a straightened leg, and exhale with the ease of a gentle bend. Let your breath dance in rhythm with your movements.

Safety Tips: If anything feels uneasy, adjust the distance from the wall or modify the motion. Your safety takes center stage.

Engaged Body Parts: Sense the strength in your grounded foot, the stretch in your extended leg, and the stability in your hips.

23. Arms Overhead

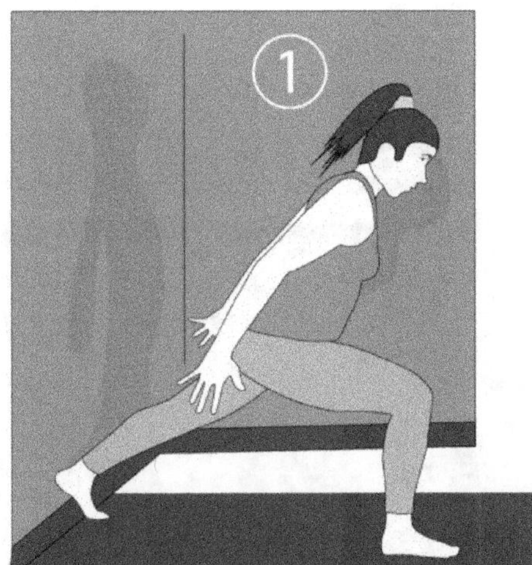 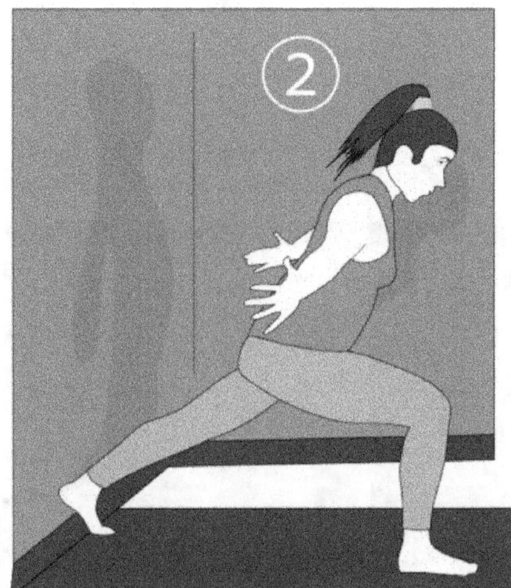 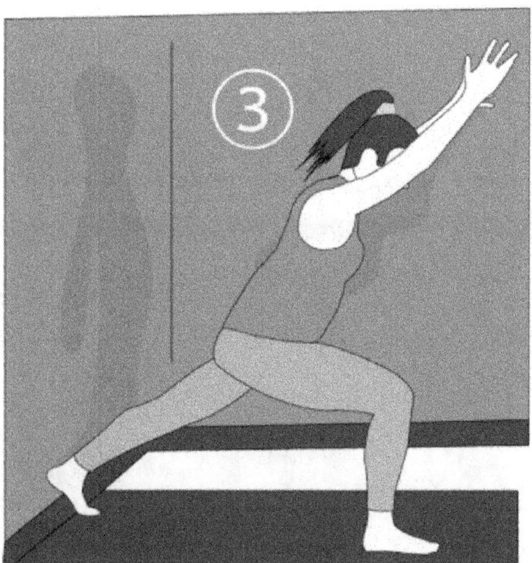

- Stand with the wall behind you, about an arm's length away.

- Position your hands behind you in a diagonal line, inward-facing, shoulder-distance apart. (1)

- Bend your right knee deeply, almost reaching a 90-degree angle, and keep your left leg straight with the calf against the wall. Ensure your right foot stays firmly on the ground. (2)

- From this grounded stance, smoothly lift your arms overhead, facing inward. Repeat this motion 10 times for a refreshing stretch. Then, switch legs. (3)

Body Awareness Tips: Pay attention to the openness in your chest and shoulders as you extend your arms overhead. Feel the gentle stretch along your side and the engagement in your leg muscles.

Breath Tips: Inhale as you prepare for the movement, and exhale as you reach your arms overhead. Let your breath guide the flow of the exercise, promoting relaxation.

Safety Tips: Keep the movement controlled and within a comfortable range. If you experience any strain, consider adjusting the depth of your knee bend. Listen to your body and move at a pace that feels right for you.

Engaged Body Parts: Sense the strength in your supporting leg, especially the muscles around your knee and thigh. Feel the stretch in your chest and shoulders as your arms move overhead, engaging your upper body.

24. Shoulder Stretch

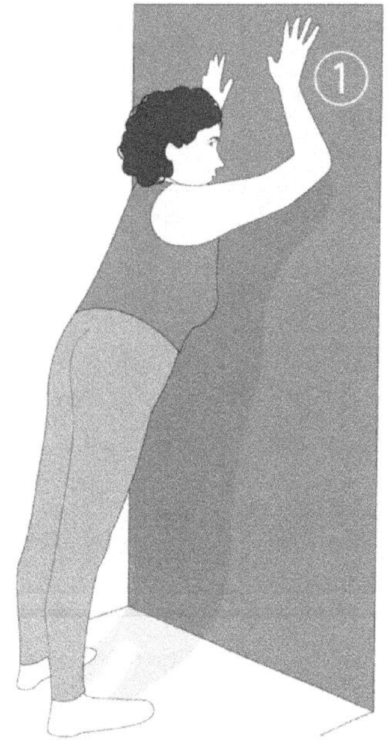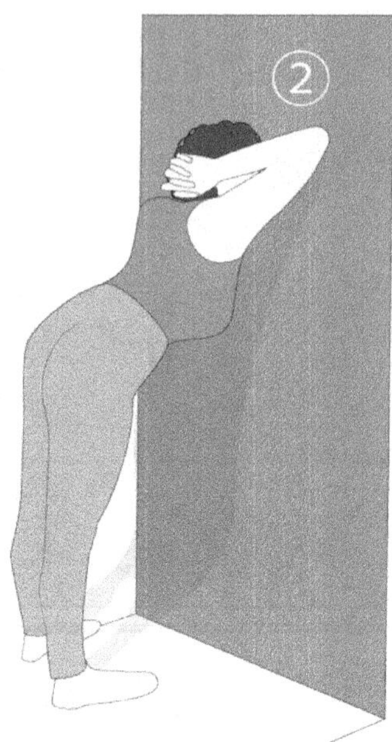

- Step into a moment of self-care as you face the wall, maintaining a comfortable 20-inch distance.

- Gently lean your chest forward, allowing your forearms to find a cozy spot on the wall. (1)

- Now, intertwine your fingers behind your neck and let your forearms press into the wall, guiding you into a soothing closeness. (2)

- Feel the stretch embracing your entire upper body, bringing your chin as close to the wall as it feels right.

Body Awareness Tips: Tune into the intricate symphony of sensations as your chest, shoulders, and neck gracefully participate in this rejuvenating stretch.

Breath Tips: Inhale the tranquility of the stretch, exhale any lingering tension. Let your breath be a gentle guide, accompanying each inch closer to the wall.

Safety Tips: Embrace comfort over intensity. If any part of the stretch feels too much, ease back. Your body sets the pace, ensuring a safe and enjoyable experience.

Engaged Body Parts: Sense the delightful opening in your chest and shoulders, the lengthening in your spine, and the subtle engagement in your neck.

25. Calf Activation

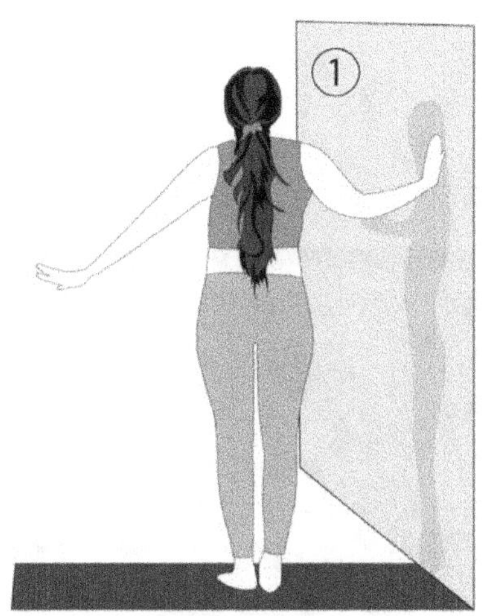 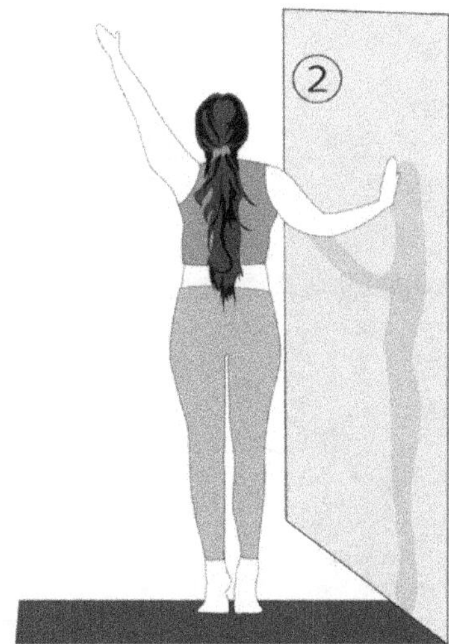

- Find your space parallel to the wall, your right hand casually resting against it and the left arm draped across your side. Feet together, preparing for a refreshing calf activation. (1)

- As you inhale deeply, gracefully raise your left arm with the palm facing inward, lifting both calves off the floor simultaneously. (2)

- Exhale slowly as you lower your calves, inch by inch, returning to the ground. Repeat this invigorating movement about 10 times, then switch sides for a balanced experience.

Body Awareness Tips: Tune into the lively sensations in your calves and the easy alignment of your body parallel to the wall. Feel the gentle stretch along your side as your arm gracefully rises.

Breath Tips: Inhale the freshness of the moment as you lift, and exhale with a sense of ease as you gently lower. Keep your breath steady and in harmony with your movements.

Safety Tips: Keep a stable and comfortable stance, avoiding any strain on your lower back or calves. If you sense any discomfort, consider adjusting the range of your motion to suit your body's rhythm.

Engaged Body Parts: Direct your focus to the vibrant activation in your calves, savoring the subtle engagement in your arm and relishing the stretch along your side.

Chapter 7: Advance Wall Pilates Exercises

In this Chapter, we delve into a series of challenging yet rewarding wall-based exercises tailored for those seeking an advanced Pilates experience.
Get ready to explore a new dimension of Wall Pilates, where precision meets intensity, and each movement is a step toward mastery.

Let's embark on this exciting Chapter together and take your Wall Pilates expertise to greater heights!

1. Wall-Extended Cow-Cat Stretch

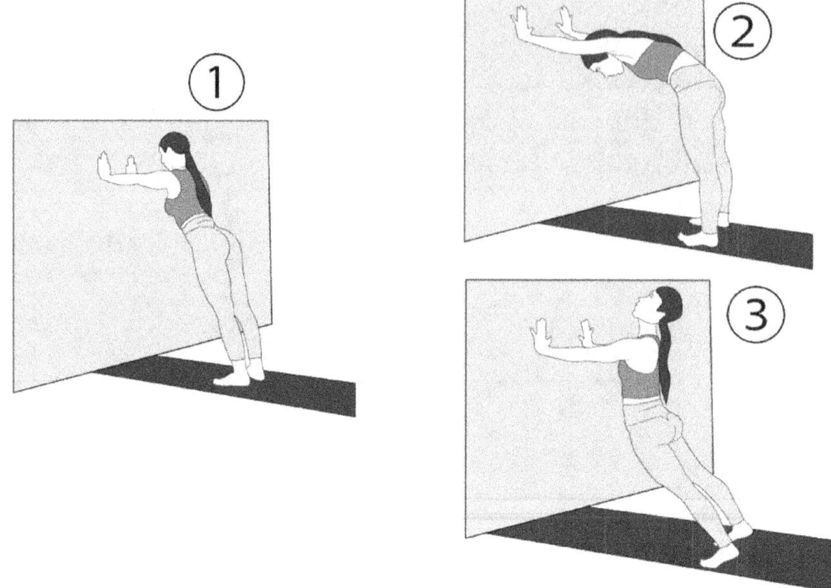

- Begin by facing the wall, standing at a distance with your feet hip-width apart, and arms extended straight, hands placed against the wall at shoulder height. (1) Ensure your arms are parallel to the ground and your body is in a straight line.

- Inhale as you initiate the movement by arching your back and bringing your chest and abdomen closer to the wall. Lift your gaze upward, allowing your spine to extend in the cow position. (2)

- Exhale as you reverse the movement. Round your back by pushing your hands into the wall and tucking your chin to your chest. Feel the stretch along your spine in the cat position. (3)

- Repeat the sequence 5 times, flowing smoothly between cow and cat stretches.

Body Awareness Tips: Focus on the sensation of your spine moving through each position, from extension to flexion.

Breath Tips: Inhale during the cow stretch, exhale during the cat stretch, and maintain a steady and controlled breath.

Safety Tips: Keep your movements within a comfortable range, and ensure your arms are at a height that allows for a smooth transition.

Engaged Body Parts: Activate your core muscles to support the movement and feel the stretch along your spine, shoulders, and chest.

2. Wall Supported Leg Lifts

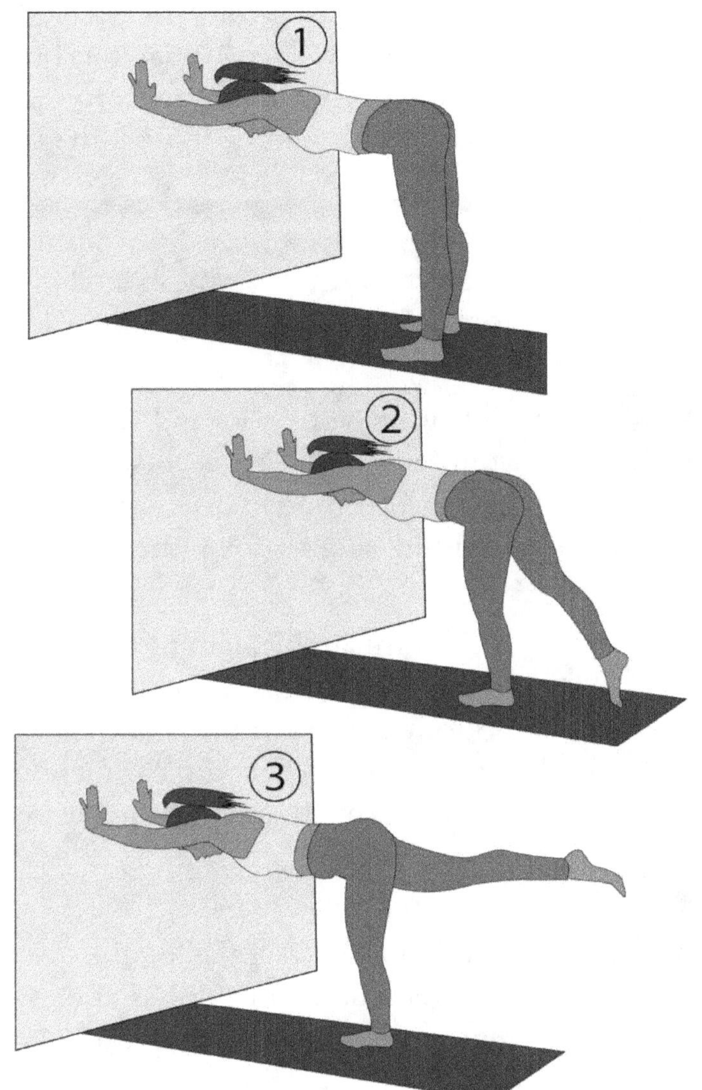

- Stand facing the wall and place your hands on it, arms extended at shoulder height. Ensure your body is in a stable position, with feet hip-width apart. (1)

- Begin by lifting your right leg straight back, keeping it parallel to the floor. Maintain a straight torso, avoiding any rotation or tilting. (2)

- Hold the position for a moment, feeling the engagement in your glutes and the back of your leg. (3)

- Lower your right leg back and repeat the movement on the left side, lifting the left leg straight back.

Body Awareness Tips: Pay attention to maintaining a straight and stable torso, avoiding any twisting or leaning.

Breath Tips: Inhale as you prepare, exhale as you lift each leg, and inhale as you lower it back down.

Safety Tips: Keep a slight bend in your standing knee for added stability, and ensure your hands are securely placed on the wall.

Engaged Body Parts: Feel the activation in your core, glutes, and the muscles of the lifted leg.

3. Wall Squat with Arm Extension

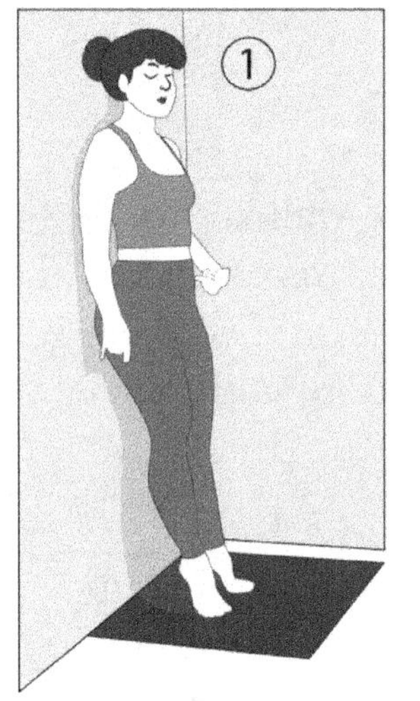

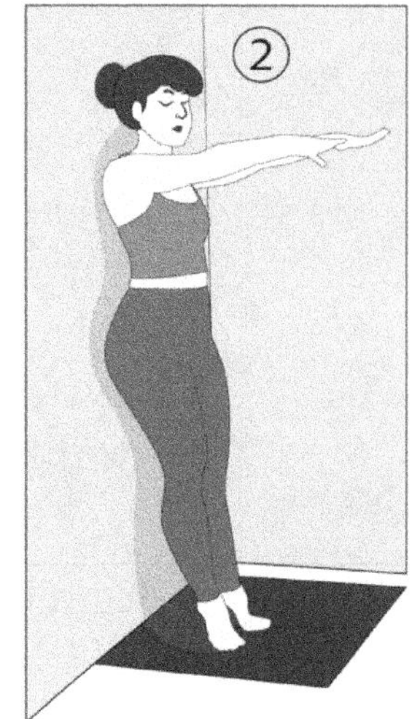

- Start standing with your back against the wall, ensuring your butt is about 3-4 inches away from it. Your feet should be hip-width apart (1)

- Start with your arms extended forward, parallel to the floor. (2)

- Engage your core and ensure your back is resting against the wall. Lower your body into a squat position, sliding down the wall. (3)

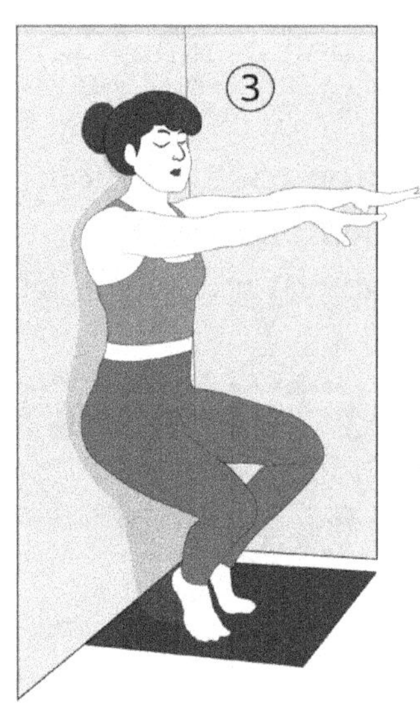

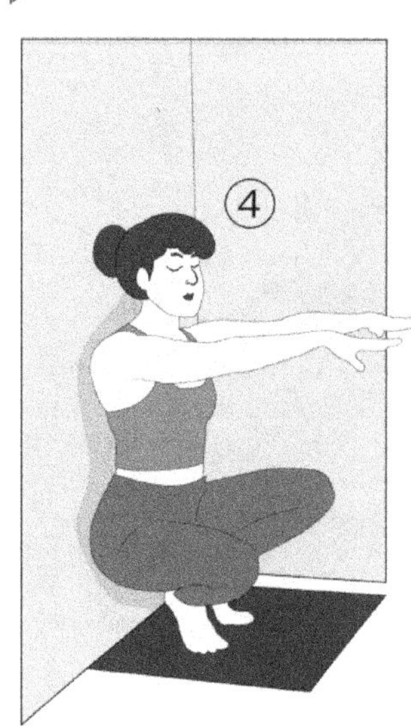

- If comfortable, aim to bend your legs deeply, almost touching your bottom to the floor. Keep your arms extended forward throughout the squat, maintaining shoulder height. (4)

- Hold the squat, feeling the engagement in your thighs and glutes. Carefully rise back up.

Body Awareness Tips: Focus on maintaining alignment and feeling the engagement in your thighs and glutes.

Breath Tips: Inhale as you prepare for the squat, exhale as you lower down, and inhale as you rise back up.

Safety Tips: If you have knee concerns, adjust the depth of the squat to a comfortable level. Listen to your body and avoid pushing into discomfort.

Engaged Body Parts: Feel the activation in your thighs, glutes, and the muscles of your core.

4. Kneeling Wall Supported Leg Lifts

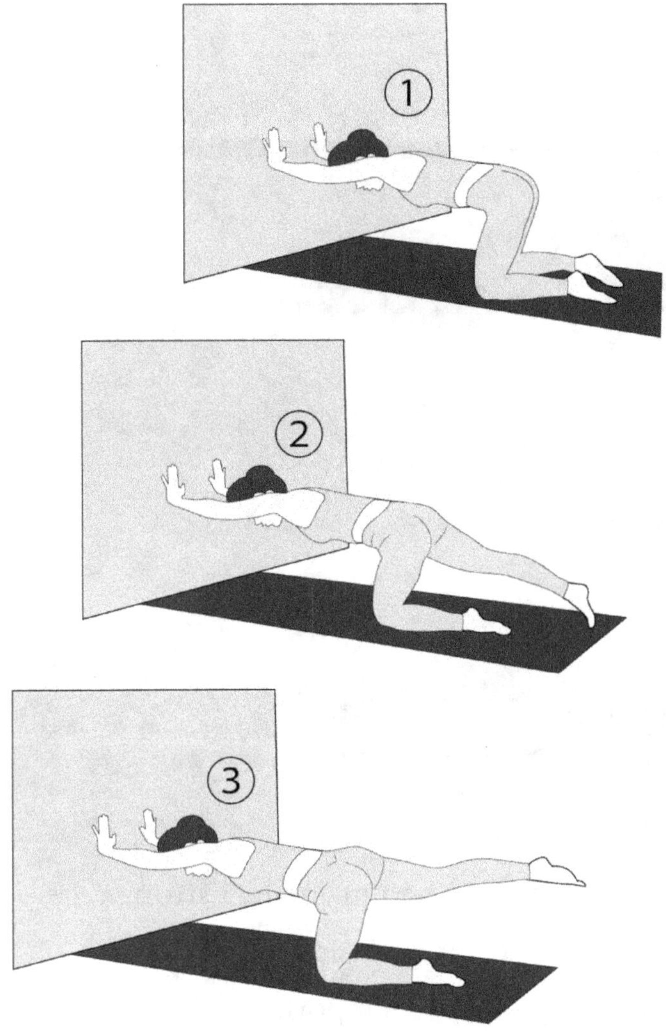

- Kneel facing the wall with your hands on it, arms extended at shoulder height. Ensure your body is in a stable position, with knees hip-width apart. (1)

- Begin by lifting your right leg straight back, keeping it parallel to the floor. Maintain a straight torso, avoiding any rotation or tilting. (2)

- Hold the position for a moment, feeling the engagement in your glutes and the back of your leg. (3)

- Lower your right leg back, then repeat the movement on the left side, lifting the left leg straight back.

Body Awareness Tips: Pay attention to maintaining a straight and stable torso, avoiding any twisting or leaning.

Breath Tips: Inhale as you prepare, exhale as you lift each leg, and inhale as you lower it back down.

Safety Tips: Keep a slight bend in your kneeling knee for added stability, and ensure your hands are securely placed on the wall.

Engaged Body Parts: **Feel** the activation in your core, glutes, and the muscles of the lifted leg.

5. Extended Wall Bridge

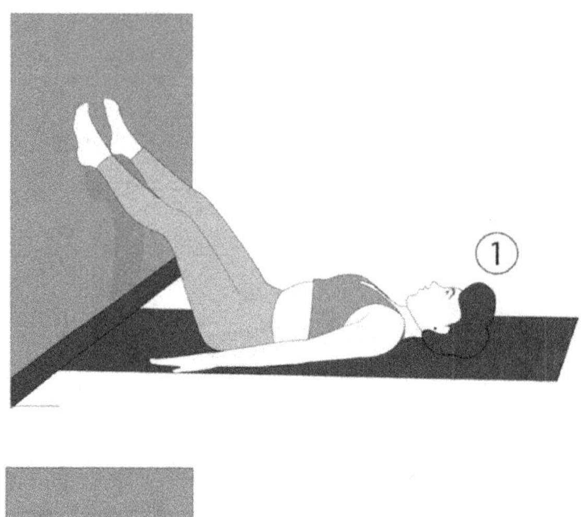

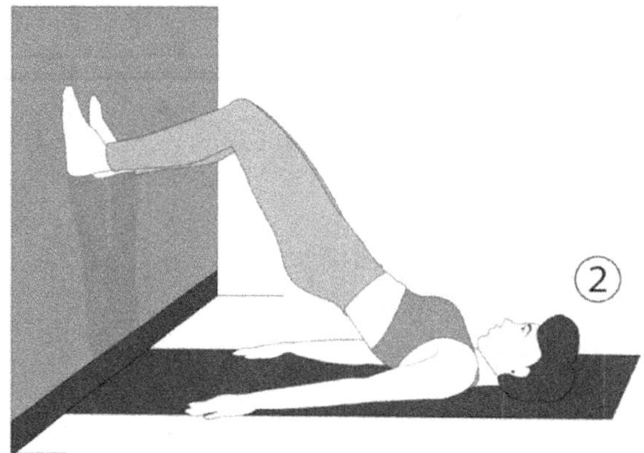

- Lie on your back with your legs slightly bent against the wall.
- Engage your core, lift your hips towards the ceiling, and maintain a strong core.
- Maintain for 1 minute at least, then lower and rest for 30 seconds.
- You can also bring your hands to your glutes for extra support.
- Repeat 5 times.

Body Awareness Tips: Focus on maintaining alignment and feeling the engagement in your core.

Breath Tips: Inhale as you prepare, exhale as you lift, and inhale on the way down.

Safety Tips: Ensure that you are comfortable and avoid straining your neck.

Engaged Body Parts: The core, glutes, and thighs are actively involved.

Chapter 8: 28-Day Wall Pilates Workout Plan

Welcome to Chapter 8 of our Wall Pilates journey! In this chapter, we present a structured and invigorating 28-day Wall Pilates Workout Plan designed to elevate your practice. With just 15 minutes a day, this plan is crafted to seamlessly integrate into your routine while delivering effective results.

Each day, you'll find a detailed plan specifying the exercises to perform, their duration, and the corresponding stretches. In addition, for each day, you will find:

- Today's focus;
- 1 breathing technique (1 minute), to perform at the beginning of the routine;
- 2 warm-up exercises (2 minutes);
- The workout for a maximum of 10 minutes - make sure to perform each pose as illustrated in the chapters;
- 2 cool-down exercises (2 minutes).

Also, the provided tracking template allows you to monitor your progress day by day, which makes it easier to stay grounded and committed to your wellness goals.

Prepare to embark on a transformative 28-day experience that not only strengthens your body but also enhances your connection with Wall Pilates. Let's dive into this purposeful plan, one day at a time ;)

Day	Focus	Breath Technique	Warm-Up	Workout	Cool-Down
1	Basics	Bellows Breathing (1 min)	Wall Roll and Stretch (Ch 3; Pose 1), Hip-Opener Leverage (Ch 3; Pose 2)	**Foundation Training Bridge (Ch 6; Pose 12),** Legs in the Sky (Ch 6; Pose 6), **Wall Push-Up to Plank (Ch 5; Pose 1),** Forearm Push-Up (Ch 5; Pose 4), **Point Your Toes (Ch 6; Pose 3)**	Seated Forward Bend (Ch 3; Pose 4), Butterfly Stretch (Ch 3; Pose 3)
2	Core	Diaphragmatic Breathing (1 min)	Cactus Arms (Ch 6; Pose16), Swing and Stretch (Ch 3; Pose 3)	**Half Arms-Wheel (Ch 6; Pose 2),** Wall-Sitting with Raised Knees (Ch 6; Pose 13), **Arms Overhead (Ch 6; Pose 23),** Wall Curl with Leg Extension (Ch 5; Pose 6), **Wall Reverse Twist Crunch (Ch 5; Pose 7),** Wall-Plow Pose (Ch 6; Pose 10)	Side Bend (Ch 6; Pose 14), Shoulder Stretch (Ch 6; Pose 24)
3	Dynamic Balance	Box Breathing (1 min)	Straight and Bent (Ch 6; Pose 22), Legs Circles (Ch 6; Pose 8)	**Legs in the Sky (Ch 6; Pose 6),** Legs in the Sky 90 Degrees (Ch 6; Pose 7), **180 Degrees (Ch 6; Pose 17),** Point Your Toes (Ch 6; Pose 3)	Seated Forward Bend (Ch 3; Pose 4), Foundation Training Bridge (Ch 6; Pose 12)

Day	Focus	Breath Technique	Warm-Up	Workout	Cool-Down
4	Energize	Lateral Breathing (1 min)	Arms Movements (Ch 6; Pose4), Legs in the Sky (Ch 6; Pose 6)	**Wall Slide and Squat (Ch 5; Pose 5),** Bridge Pose with Bent Knees (Ch 6; Pose 1), **Forearm Plank with Feet on the Wall (Ch 6; Pose 5),** Push-up Internal Hands Rotation (Ch 6; Pose 19), **Wall Push-Up to Plank (Ch 5; Pose 1)**	Seated Opposing Toe-Tapping (Ch 3; Pose 1), Butterfly Stretch (Ch 3; Pose 3)
5	Power	Diaphrag matic Breathing (1 min)	Wall Push-Up to Plank (Ch 5; Pose 1), Standing Wall Slide-Down (Ch 5; Pose 2)	**Bridge Pose with Straight Legs (Ch 6; Pose 9),** Half Arms-Wheel (Ch 6; Pose 2), **Wall Curl with Leg Extension (Ch 5; Pose 6),** Wall Squat With Cushion Squeeze (Ch 5; Pose 3), **Hand on the Back of the Head (Ch 6; Pose 20)**	Seated Forward Bend (Ch 3; Pose 4), Wall-Plow Pose (Ch 6; Pose 10)
6	Flexibility	Lateral Breathing (1 min)	Legs in the Sky 90 Degrees (Ch 6; Pose 7), Active Calf Release (Ch 3; Pose 4)	**Forearm Push-Up (Ch 5; Pose 4),** Push-ups with Internal Hands Rotation (Ch 6; Pose 19), **Calf Activation (Ch 6; Pose 25),** Arms Overhead (Ch 6; Pose 23)	Side Bend (Ch 6; Pose 14), Shoulder Stretch (Ch 6; Pose 24)

Day	Focus	Breath Technique	Warm-Up	Workout	Cool-Down
7	Core	Box Breathing (1 min)	Swing and Stretch (Ch 3; Pose 3), Point Your Toes (Ch 6; Pose 3)	**Straight and Bent (Ch 6; Pose 22),** Cactus Arms (Ch 6; Pose 16), **Legs Circles (Ch 6; Pose 8),** Hand on the Back of the Head (Ch 6; Pose 20)	Foundation Training Bridge (Ch 6; Pose 12), Butterfly Stretch (Ch 3; Pose 3)
8	Strength	Bellows Breathing (1 min)	Straight and Bent (Ch 6; Pose22), Hand on the Back of the Head (Ch 6; Pose20)	**Bridge Pose with Bent Knees (Ch 6; Pose 1),** Legs in the Sky 90 Degrees (Ch 6; Pose 7), **Wall Reverse Twist Crunch (Ch 5; Pose 7),** Wall Supported Leg Lifts (Ch 7; Pose 2), **Extended Wall Bridge (Ch 7; Pose 5)**	Wall-Plow Pose (Ch 6; Pose 10), Seated Forward Bent (Ch 3; Pose 4)
9	Balance	Diaphragmatic Breathing (1 min)	Legs Circles (Ch 6; Pose 8), Arms Movements (Ch 6; Pose 4)	**Legs in the Sky (Ch 6; Pose 6),** Wall Push-Up to Plank (Ch 5; Pose 1), **180 Degrees (Ch 6; Pose 17),** Push-ups with Internal Hands Rotation (Ch 6; Pose 19)	Straight and Bent (Ch 6; Pose 22), Point Your Toes (Ch 6; Pose 3)

Day	Focus	Breath Technique	Warm-Up	Workout	Cool-Down
10	Total Body	Diaphragmatic Breathing (1 min)	Tap the Toes (Ch 6; Pose 21), Legs in the Sky (Ch 6; Pose 6)	**Bridge Pose with Straight Legs (Ch 6; Pose 9),** Half Arms-Wheel (Ch 6; Pose 2), **Legs Circles (Ch 6; Pose 8),** Wall Reverse Twist Crunch (Ch 5; Pose 7), **Hand on the Back of the Head (Ch 6; Pose 20)**	Seated Spinal Twist (Ch 3; Pose 2), Foundation Training Bridge (Ch 6; Pose 12)
11	Power	Lateral Breathing (1 min)	Wall Roll and Stretch (Ch 3; Pose 1), Tap the Toes (Ch 6; Pose 21)	**Legs Circles (Ch 6; Pose 8),** Forearm Plank with Feet on the Wall (Ch 6; Pose 5), **Wall Squat with Arm Extension (Ch 7; Pose 3),** 180 Reverse (Ch 6; Pose 18), **Hand on the Back of the Head (Ch 6; Pose 20)**	Seated Opposing Toe-Tapping (Ch 3; Pose 1), Seated Spinal Twist (Ch 3; Pose 2)
12	Core	Bellows Breathing (1 min)	Legs in the Sky (Ch 6; Pose6), Cactus Arms (Ch 6; Pose 16)	**Bridge Pose with Bent Knees (Ch 6; Pose 1),** Legs in the Sky 90 Degrees (Ch 6; Pose 7), **Wall Supported Leg Lifts (Ch 7; Pose 2),** Push-ups with Internal Hands Rotation (Ch 6; Pose 19), **Arms Overhead (Ch 6; Pose 23)**	Shoulder Stretch (Ch 6; Pose 24), Seated Spinal Twist (Ch 3; Pose 2)

Day	Focus	Breath Technique	Warm-Up	Workout	Cool-Down
13	Glutes	Diaphragmatic Breathing (1 min)	Straight and Bent (Ch 6; Pose22), Legs Circles (Ch 6; Pose 8)	**Legs in the Sky (Ch 6; Pose 6),** Point Your Toes (Ch 6; Pose 3), **Kneeling Wall Supported Leg Lifts (Ch 7; Pose 4),** Wall Squat with Arm Extension (Ch 7; Pose 3), **Wall-Plow Pose (Ch 6; Pose 10)**	Seated Opposing Toe-Tapping (Ch 3; Pose 1), Seated Forward Bend (Ch 3; Pose 4)
14	Flexibility & Concentration	Box Breathing (1 min)	Arms Overhead (Ch 6; Pose 23), Arms Movements (Ch 6; Pose 4)	**Push-up Internal Hands Rotation (Ch 6; Pose 19),** Bridge Pose with Straight Legs (Ch 6; Pose 9), **Calf Activation (Ch 6; Pose 25),** Hand on the Back of the Head (Ch 6; Pose 20)	Side Bend (Ch 6; Pose 14), Shoulder Stretch (Ch 6; Pose 24)
15	Upper & Lower Body	Bellows Breathing (1 min)	Tap the Toes (Ch 6; Pose21), Active Calf Release (Ch 3; Warm-up Pose 4)	**Legs Circles (Ch 6; Pose 8),** 180 Degrees (Ch 6; Pose 17), **Wall Push-Up to Plank (Ch 5; Pose 1),** Arms Overhead (Ch 6; Pose 23)	Foundation Training Bridge (Ch 6; Pose 12), Butterfly Stretch (Ch 3; Pose 3)

Day	Focus	Breath Technique	Warm-Up	Workout	Cool-Down
16	Deep Awakening	Diaphragmatic Breathing (1 min)	Cactus Arms (Ch 6; Pose16), Swing and Stretch (Ch 3; Pose3)	**Bridge Pose with Bent Knees (Ch 6; Pose1),** Point Your Toes (Ch 6; Pose 3), **Foundation Training Bridge (Ch 6; Pose 12),** Legs Circles (Ch 6; Pose 8), **Tap the Toes (Ch 6; Pose 21)**	Seated Forward Bend (Ch 3; Pose 4), Shoulder Stretch (Ch 6; Pose 24)
17	Full Body Harmony	Lateral Breathing (1 min)	Legs in the Sky (Ch 6; Pose 6), Half Arms-Wheel (Ch 6; Pose 2)	**Forearm Plank with Feet on the Wall (Ch 6; Pose 5),** Hand on the Back of the Head (Ch 6; Pose 20), **Arms Overhead (Ch 6; Pose 23),** 180 Reverse (Ch 6; Pose 18), **Calf Activation (Ch 6; Pose 25),** Straight and Bent (Ch 6; Pose 22)	Legs Circles (Ch 6; Pose 8), Cactus Arms (Ch 6; Pose 16)
18	Core	Diaphragmatic Breathing (1 min)	Legs in the Sky 90 Degrees (Ch 6; Pose 7), Swing and Stretch (Ch 3; Pose 3)	**Bridge Pose with Straight Legs (Ch 6; Pose 9),** Half Arms-Wheel (Ch 6; Pose 2), **Legs Circles (Ch 6; Pose 8),** Foundation Training Bridge (Ch 6; Pose 12), **Tap the Toes (Ch 6; Pose 21)**	Seated Forward Fold (Ch 6; Pose 15), Shoulder Stretch (Ch 6; Pose 24)

Day	Focus	Breath Technique	Warm-Up	Workout	Cool-Down
19	Upper Body	Box Breathing (1 min)	Arms Movements (Ch 6; Pose4), Seated Forward Fold (Ch 6; Pose15)	**Push-ups with Internal Hands Rotation (Ch 6; Pose 19),** Hand on the Back of the Head (Ch 6; Pose 20), **180 Degrees (Ch 6; Pose 17),** 180 Reverse (Ch 6; Pose 18), **Shoulder Stretch (Ch 6; Pose 24),** Calf Activation (Ch 6; Pose 25)	Butterfly Stretch (Ch 3; Pose 3), Seated Forward Bend (Ch 3; Pose 4)
20	Balance & Core	Lateral Breathing (1 min)	Wall-Plow Pose (Ch 6; Pose10), Swing and Stretch (Ch 3; Warm-up Pose 3)	**Legs in the Sky (Ch 6; Pose 6),** Bridge Pose with Bent Knees (Ch 6; Pose 1), **Point Your Toes (Ch 6; Pose 3),** Half Arms-Wheel (Ch 6; Pose 2), **Hand on the Back of the Head (Ch 6; Pose 20)**	Seated Forward Fold (Ch 6; Pose 15), Legs Circles (Ch 6; Pose 8)
21	Total Body	Bellows Breathing (1 min)	Tap the Toes (Ch 6; Pose21), Seated Forward Fold (Ch 6; Pose15)	**Legs Circles (Ch 6; Pose 18),** Wall Push-Up to Plank (Ch 5; Pose 1), **Wall Squat With Cushion Squeeze (Ch 5; Pose 3),** Point Your Toes (Ch 6; Pose 3), **Wall-Plow Pose (Ch 6; Pose 10)**	Cactus Arms (Ch 6; Pose 16), Tilt Forward (Ch 6; Pose 11)

Day	Focus	Breath Technique	Warm-Up	Workout	Cool-Down
22	Strength	Diaphragmatic Breathing (1 min)	Legs in the Sky 90 Degrees (Ch 6; Pose 7), Standing Wall Slide-Down (Ch 5; Pose 2)	**Bridge Pose with Straight Legs (Ch 6; Pose 8),** Half Arms-Wheel (Ch 6; Pose 2), **Forearm Plank with Feet on the Wall (Ch 6; Pose 5),** Calf Activation (Ch 6; Pose 25), **Forearm Push-Up (Ch 5; Pose 4),** Foundation Training Bridge (Ch 6; Pose 12)	Seated Forward Fold (Ch 6; Pose 15), Legs Circles (Ch 6; Pose 8)
23	Harmony	Bellows Breathing (1 min)	Arms Movements (Ch 6; Pose 4), Hip-Opener Leverage (Ch 3; Pose 2)	**Push-up Internal Hands Rotation (Ch 6; Pose 19),** Hand on the Back of the Head (Ch 6; Pose 20), **180 Degrees (Ch 6; Pose 17),** Shoulder Stretch (Ch 6; Pose 24), **Straight and Bent (Ch 6; Pose 22)**	Legs in the Sky (Ch 6; Pose 6), Cactus Arms (Ch 6; Pose 16)
24	Mind & Concentration	Box Breathing (1 min)	Wall-Plow Pose (Ch 6; Pose 10), Half Arms-Wheel (Ch 6; Pose 2)	**Legs in the Sky (Ch 6; Pose 6),** Bridge Pose with Bent Knees (Ch 6; Pose 1), **Point Your Toes (Ch 6; Pose 3),** Legs Circles (Ch 6; Pose 8), **Wall-Extended Cow-Cat Stretch (Ch 7; Pose 1)**	Seated Forward Fold (Ch 6; Pose 15), Shoulder Stretch (Ch 6; Pose 24)

Day	Focus	Breath Technique	Warm-Up	Workout	Cool-Down
25	Upper and Lower Body	Lateral Breathing (1 min)	Arms Overhead (Ch 6; Pose23), Wall Roll and Stretch (Ch 3; Warm-up Pose 1)	**Wall Push-Up to Plank (Ch 5; Pose 1),** Wall Squat with Arm Extension (Ch 7; Pose 3), **Calf Activation (Ch 6; Pose 25),** Point Your Toes (Ch 6; Pose 3), **Forearm Plank with Feet on the Wall (Ch 6; Pose 5)**	Tilt Forward (Ch 6; Pose 11), Foundation Training Bridge (Ch 6; Pose 12)
26	Core	Diaphragmatic Breathing (1 min)	Wall-Extended Cow-Cat Stretch (Ch 7; Pose 1), Cactus Arms (Ch 6; Pose16)	**Bridge Pose with Bent Knees (Ch 6; Pose 1),** Point Your Toes (Ch 6; Pose 3), **Extended Wall Bridge (Ch 7; Pose 5),** Legs Circles (Ch 6; Pose 8), **Tap the Toes (Ch 6; Pose 21)**	Shoulder Stretch (Ch 6; Pose 24), Seated Spinal Twist (Ch 3; Cool Down Pose 2)
27	Full Body	Lateral Breathing (1 min)	Legs in the Sky (Ch 6; Pose 6), Arms Overhead (Ch 6; Pose23)	**Forearm Plank with Feet on the Wall (Ch 6; Pose 5),** Hand on the Back of the Head (Ch 6; Pose 20), **Wall Squat With Cushion Squeeze (Ch 5; Pose 3),** Calf Activation (Ch 6; Pose 25), **Forearm Push-Up (Ch 5; Pose 4)**	Legs Circles (Ch 6; Pose 8), Cactus Arms (Ch 6; Pose 16)

Day	Focus	Breath Technique	Warm-Up	Workout	Cool-Down
28	Grand Finale	Bellow Breathing (1 min)	Seated Forward Fold (Ch 6; Pose15), Tap the Toes (Ch 6; Pose21)	**Legs Circles (Ch 6; Pose 8),** Wall Push-Up to Plank (Ch 5; Pose 1), **Standing Wall Slide-Down (Ch 5; Pose 2),** Arms Overhead (Ch 6; Pose 23), **Point Your Toes (Ch 6; Pose 3)**	Wall-Plow Pose (Ch 6; Pose 10), Tilt Forward (Ch 6; Pose 11)

Chapter 9: Final Tips on Cultivating a Healthy Lifestyle

As we have said so many times already, the Wall Pilates journey is not just about movements; it's about transforming your lifestyle. In the last Chapter, we will explore some crucial tips to cultivate a holistic sense of well-being.

Integrated Wellness Approach

Consider Wall Pilates as more than just a workout routine. It's a puzzle piece in your larger health canvas.

- Explore the synergies between mindful movements against the wall, nourishing your body with wholesome nutrition, and cultivating mental resilience.

- Understand how each session of Wall Pilates contributes not only to physical strength but also to mental clarity, creating a harmonious balance that extends beyond the boundaries of traditional fitness routines.

- Incorporate nutrition as a complementary force, fueling your body for the demands of Wall Pilates. Delve into the symbiotic relationship where the proper nutrients enhance your performance and recovery, creating a holistic foundation for overall well-being. Embrace the mindful nourishment that echoes the precision and intentionality of your Wall Pilates practice - you will discover that in your '6 Dietary Tips' e-book!

- Wall Pilates is a sanctuary for mental well-being, where the rhythmic flow of movements becomes a form of meditation. In this fusion of physical activity, nutrition, and mental wellness, Wall Pilates emerges as a transformative practice that nurtures the entirety of your well-being.

Quality Rest and Recovery

Quality rest and recovery are essential components of a well-rounded health and fitness plan, including the practice of Wall Pilates. In the pursuit of a healthier lifestyle, the emphasis often falls on physical activity and nutrition, but the role of rest and recovery should not be underestimated. Here are some tips:

Mindful Wind-Down Session: As part of your bedtime routine, engage in a mindful wind-down session before hitting the hay. Incorporate gentle Wall Pilates stretches that focus on releasing tension in critical areas such as the neck, shoulders, and lower back. This deliberate movement helps signal to your body that it's time to relax and prepares your mind for a peaceful night's sleep.

Some suggestions for choosing the stretches:
- Chapter 3; Cool-Down Pose no.3, Butterfly Stretch.
- Chapter 3; Cool-Down Pose no.4, Seated Forward Bend.
- Chapter 4; Breathing Technique no.2, Lateral Breathing.
- Charter 5; Pose no.6, Wall Curl with Leg Extension (no curl, only rest with legs at the wall).
- Chapter 6; Pose no. 15, Seated Forward Fold.
- Chapter 6; Pose no. 16, Cactus Arms.

Breathwork for Serenity: Integrate calming breathwork exercises into your pre-sleep ritual. Explore deep diaphragmatic breathing (Chapter 4; Breathing Technique no.1) with your back against the wall, allowing your breath to guide you into a tranquil state. Wall Pilates offers excellent support for these practices, fostering a sense of calm and helping you transition smoothly into a restful slumber.

Screen-Free Zone: Establish a screen-free zone at least an hour before bedtime. Instead of scrolling through electronic devices, spend this time engaging in a Wall Pilates routine that promotes gentle movement and mindfulness. The absence of screens contributes to a healthier sleep environment, enhancing your body's natural circadian rhythm.

Create a Restful Atmosphere: Craft a soothing bedtime ambiance by dimming the lights and incorporating relaxing elements into your space. After your Wall Pilates routine, indulge in a warm, calming beverage like herbal tea or camomille. As you wind down, savor the tranquility and let the Wall Pilates experience guide you into a restorative night of sleep.

Integrate a Rest Day: Recognize the importance of rest days in your fitness routine. While Wall Pilates can invigorate your body, allowing it time to rest is equally vital. Consider incorporating a designated rest day to recharge, allowing your muscles to recover and ensuring a holistic approach to your well-being.

Building a Support System

Connecting with the Wall Pilates community can amplify your experiences and keep you motivated. That's why it's pivotal to boost motivation and fun during this journey!

Sharing experiences, progress, and challenges with others who are on a similar fitness journey (even family members or friends), in fact, can significantly enhance your own motivation and enjoyment. Pilates, like any form of exercise, can sometimes feel like an individual pursuit. However, when you engage with a community of like-minded individuals, it becomes a shared experience.
This not only makes the process more enjoyable but also helps overcome potential hurdles. The encouragement and shared experiences within the community can turn the pursuit of health into a collective and uplifting endeavor, amplifying the overall satisfaction and motivation during your Wall Pilates journey.

As we wrap up, remember that Wall Pilates isn't a mere workout; it's a lifestyle. It's about nurturing your body, mind, and soul. So, let's dive into these final insights and pave the way for a healthier, more balanced you.

Conclusion: Wall Pilates Holistic Wellness

As we wrap up our journey through Wall Pilates, I want to leave you with some key takeaways. This exploration has been more than just a guide to physical exercises; it's been a pathway to a holistic lifestyle intertwining with your overall well-being.

Let's talk about the silent force at the core of Wall Pilates – the breath. Throughout our discussions, we've uncovered the significance of conscious breathing, discovering techniques that not only energize the body during workouts but also cleanse the mind, inducing a sense of calm. This understanding of breath mechanics isn't confined to Pilates; it's a tool for daily life, offering benefits far beyond the boundaries of a workout.

Our exploration also delved into exercises targeting various muscle groups, revealing the importance of mindful movement and core engagement. From diaphragmatic breathing to lateral breathing, these foundational principles laid the groundwork for exercises that sculpt not just the body but foster a profound connection between mind and muscle. Pilates isn't merely a physical workout; it's a cognitive journey demanding focus, precision, and control.

Beyond the mat, we've explored how Wall Pilates seamlessly integrates with daily life. Whether standing against the wall, engaging in a breathing exercise, or performing dynamic movements, Pilates principles serve as a guide for cultivating awareness, promoting relaxation, and fostering a deeper connection with our bodies. Consider each exercise as a unique note in a symphony of motion. From Wall Squats to Bridge exercises, Leg Lifts, and intricate movements like the Wall Curl with Leg Extension, we've witnessed the versatility of Pilates in building strength, flexibility, and stability. These exercises aren't mere physical tasks; they are opportunities to tune into our bodies, breathing life into each movement with intention.

The 28-day workout plan, requiring just 15 minutes a day, demonstrated the practical application of Wall Pilates. It's not just about the exercises; it's about consistency, progression, and self-discovery. The tracking template provided a roadmap, allowing us to witness growth and celebrate small victories along the way.

In the final chapters, we explored the delicate balance between physical activity, nutrition, and mental wellness. Wall Pilates isn't just a compilation of exercises; it's a lifestyle encompassing mindful movement, conscious breathing, and a supportive community.

As you close this book, consider it not an endpoint but a springboard for continued exploration and growth. Let the principles of Wall Pilates resonate in your daily life, becoming a guiding force toward a healthier, more balanced you. May your journey be filled with strength, flexibility, and the joy of mindful movement.

Your, Denise Kelley